The NDD Book

The NDD™

Book

How Nutrition Deficit Disorder Affects
Your Child's Learning, Behavior, and Health, and
What You Can Do About It—Without Drugs

William Sears, M.D.

Little, Brown and Company
New York   Boston   London

Little, Brown and Company
Hachette Book Group
237 Park Avenue, New York, NY 10017
Visit our Web site at www.HachetteBookGroup.com

First Edition: April 2009

Little, Brown and Company is a division of Hachette Book Group, Inc.
The Little, Brown name and logo are trademarks of Hachette Book Group, Inc.

Library of Congress Cataloging-in-Publication Data
Sears, William, M.D.
    The NDD book : how nutrition deficit disorder affects your child's learning, behavior,
and health, and what you can do about it — without drugs / William Sears. — 1st ed.
        p. cm.
    Includes index.
    ISBN 978-0-316-04344-1
    1. Nutrition disorders in children. 2. Nutrition disorders in children — Prevention.
3. Diet in disease. I. Title.
    RJ399.N8S43 2009
    618.92'39 — dc22   2008051302

10 9 8 7 6 5 4 3 2 1

RRD-IN

Printed in the United States of America

To my children:
James
Robert
Peter
Hayden
Erin
Matthew
Stephen
Lauren

and grandchildren:
Andrew
Alex
Joshua
Lea
Jonathan
Ashton
Morgan
Thomas

I have tried my best to protect you from NDD. I hope parents and grandparents the world over will do the same with their families.

Contents

How to Get the Most out of This Book

To get the most out of your personal NDD-prevention plan, I suggest you take advantage of the following additional resources:

The Family Nutrition Book: Everything You Need to Know About Feeding Your Children — From Birth Through Adolescence

The Healthiest Kid in the Neighborhood: Ten Ways to Get Your Family on the Right Nutritional Track

Visit Dr. Sears online at www.AskDrSears.com to find the following:

- a free subscription to our bimonthly nutritional and parenting newsletter

- a downloadable traffic-light eating chart that you can put up on your refrigerator

- mom-to-mom moments: helpful parenting and nutritional tips from my daughter Hayden Sears-Livesay

- the food forum, an interactive blog where parents share their favorite recipes and feeding strategies, and the Drs. Sears add their comments

- our personal recommendations on nutritional supplements

- updated information from each member of the Sears team: Drs. William, Robert, James, and Peter; Hayden Sears-Livesay; and Martha Sears

A Word from Dr. Bill

Children are getting sicker, sadder, and fatter. Why? The problem is food, glorious food! During my thirty-six years as a pediatrician, I have never before seen such an epidemic of nutrition-related illnesses. In this book you will learn a new name that I have given to this epidemic: NDD, which stands for nutrition deficit disorder. The cause? Children have lost their taste for real food. The treatment? Reshape their taste back to eating real food. That's what you will learn to do in this book.

Fake food, as you will soon learn, can cause illnesses, and parents — and even many doctors — have lost sight of the fact that real food is real medicine. I will take you inside a child's brain and other body parts so that you can see how real food acts as medicine. You will learn how real food turns on the body's own internal pharmacy and how junk food interferes with the body's own natural internal medicines.

In part 1, you will learn *why* you must make changes in your family's way of eating to prevent NDD. In part 2, you will learn *how.* By following my seven steps for preventing NDD, you will be well on your way to giving your family the lifelong gift of health. To help you make NDD prevention part of your daily family living, in part 3 we will share our favorite meal plans and recipes.

I

Does Your Child Have NDD?

In this section I'll take you on a feeding trip through a child's body. You will be amazed when you see how real foods (occurring in nature) make the brain grow smarter, and fake foods (made in a factory) lead to failing grades. You will learn about a new condition, Nutrition Deficit Disorder (NDD), figure out whether your child has it, and learn how to prevent and treat it. If you are a motivated parent who already knows the connection between good eating and good health, these early chapters will reinforce your choices. If you aren't there yet, this part of the book will get you there.

1

Parents, We Have a Problem. It's NDD!

The story begins on a typical day in the office of Sears Family Pediatrics, where I have the privilege of practicing medicine with my three sons. What happened that day changed the way I practice pediatrics forever and influenced the health of hundreds of my patients. That was the day this book was born.

"Welcome to our office. How can I help you?" I greeted my first patient.

"Johnny's school thinks that he has ADD," his mother began.

"Attention deficit disorder. Hmm. . . . Tell me, what does Johnny have for breakfast?" I inquired.

"Hi-C and a Pop-Tart," Johnny's mother confessed.

"What does he have for midmorning snack?"

"Usually nothing, but sometimes he has some chips."

"What does he have for school lunch?"

"Oh, the usual pizza and stuff that kids eat."

"Johnny does not have ADD, he has NDD!" I said spontaneously, straight from my heart.

I'll never forget the surprised look on this mother's face. She

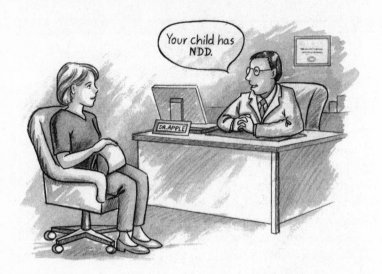

had no idea what on earth NDD was, but it sounded like something she didn't want her child to have.

"Nutrition deficit disorder," I interpreted.

I went on to explain to this puzzled parent that the brain, above all other organs, is affected, for better or worse, by what we eat. "You put junk food into a child's brain, you get back junk behavior, junk learning, and junk mood. It's as simple as that!" The mother's look of amazement immediately changed to one of comprehension. "Oh! That makes sense. I get it! NDD." Relieved, she said, "So he doesn't need drugs?"

"No, not the prescription kind. He just needs to eat real food, because real food is real medicine."

It was then that I realized that this mother, and many other moms like her, didn't understand that food can affect how her child learns, behaves, and feels.

DOES YOUR CHILD HAVE NDD?

Here are the main signs we look for when diagnosing a child with NDD:

- ☐ frequent mood swings
- ☐ unrelenting temper tantrums
- ☐ restless sleep
- ☐ poor attention span
- ☐ impulsive outbursts
- ☐ labeled with a D: ADD, ADHD, BPD, OCD, etc.
- ☐ behavior problems at school, home, and day care
- ☐ learning difficulties
- ☐ hyperactivity
- ☐ frequent infections
- ☐ dry, flaky, bumpy skin
- ☐ intestinal problems: reflux, abdominal discomforts, constipation, diarrhea
- ☐ vision problems
- ☐ frequent allergies
- ☐ dry, brittle hair
- ☐ brittle, thin nails
- ☐ very pale skin, especially on the earlobes

THE STORY OF JOHNNY

To fully understand how fake food affects a child, let's spend a day in the body and brain of a typical seven-year-old junk-food eater. Let's call him Johnny Junk-Food Eater.

Johnny awakens from a restless night's sleep. Because he went to bed with his body full of junk food, he got junk sleep. He wolfs down a junk-food breakfast and rushes off to school. Because of junk sleep and a junk breakfast, he starts his day with a big D, for being *disadvantaged*. Because he missed the head start that real food gives the brain, and the biochemical balance that real food gives the body, he enters the classroom feeling tired and with a bit of a brain fog. Johnny begins his school day with his body and brain in biochemical imbalance, so he can't keep his mind on what he is reading and what the teacher is saying.

Around nine thirty or ten, Johnny gets hungry because the fake food wasn't filling. His blood sugar drops because the junk carbs that rushed into his bloodstream at breakfast are all used up. Now he has an even harder time concentrating. Meanwhile, his brain is telling his body, "I need more fuel." So it sends a signal to his adrenal glands to pump out stress hormones, which squeeze some of the stored fuel out of his liver to feed his hungry brain. These stress hormones get Johnny hyped up, so he starts to fidget. He looks out the window because he's bored, and his stress hormones-filled body tells him, "Gotta move!" But the teacher says, "Gotta sit!" While Johnny's body sits in the classroom, his mind is already at recess. Because his brain is out of biochemical balance, so is his behavior, and he pokes the kid sitting next to him.

Around noon Johnny goes through the school lunch line for his next junk-food fix — the junk carbs and fake fats are there for the choosing. After lunch he's calmer but way too sluggish to play, which is what his body really should be doing right now. So, back to the classroom Johnny goes, with a case of double TB, *tired body* and *tired brain*. He experiences more mind wandering, more fidgeting, and more distractibility. Johnny goes home, gets a snack, and runs around outside. He feels much better for a short time. But then comes a high-carb dinner, and, naturally, both Johnny's body and brain get turned off from doing homework.

Johnny not only eats polluted food, he breathes polluted air, since his school is located near an intersection of freeways.

Because Johnny wasn't fed real food, his immune system is also out of balance. Johnny gets sick often and misses school, and this puts him further behind. His allergies flare up, too, causing him to wheeze and cough so much that his brain and body can't rest at night. The cycle continues.

Johnny gets more Ds. Of course the teacher notices that Johnny is having difficulty. To a child, being labeled *difficult* or *different* means he is less somehow — no one's fooling him — and his self-esteem goes downhill. "He's another one of those kids with ADD," the teacher concludes. "He needs medication," she tells his parents, so off to the doctor they go. What his parents don't realize is that the doctor often suffers from her own D, *distraction,* from having to see too many patients in too little time. Since the distracted doctor doesn't have enough time to take a full nutritional history, Johnny gets another D, *drugs.*

Now he starts the day with a double D, the D caused by his junk food and the D of biochemical disarray caused by the drugs. Now his body and brain are really in a metabolic mess.

Because his brain and body are out of balance, Johnny's food cravings are as well. He craves more junk food because that's what his body is used to, and this leads to overeating, which leads to weight gain. This cycle causes an even greater imbalance in body and brain and leads to more drugs.

Johnny has NDD. The rest of this book covers the changes that the parents of Johnny, who is especially junk-food-sensitive, and many other parents can make to dramatically improve their children's behavior and learning.

ONE D LEADS TO ANOTHER

Kids with one D are more likely to get other Ds because the cause is the same — nutrition deficit disorder. Children with disorders of the brain are also more likely to get diseases of the body.

The D epidemic. Parents, we have an epidemic of Ds: attention deficit disorder (ADD), obsessive compulsive disorder (OCD), autism spectrum disorder (ASD), bipolar disorder (BPD), oppositional defiant disorder (ODD), depression, and the biggest D of the decade, diabetes. To treat these Ds, children are taking more prescription drugs than ever before. While these disorders do exist and drugs are often necessary, they can be made worse and even triggered by nutrition deficit disorder. In my almost forty years as a pediatrician I have never before seen so many children get so many drugs for so many Ds. The good news is, your child does not have to be one of them. Throughout this book you will learn how to help your child dodge the Ds.

SCARY STATISTICS EVERY PARENT SHOULD PONDER

Children are getting *sicker, sadder,* and *fatter,* and NDD is responsible. Think about these alarming statistics from the past decade:

- Recently the U.S. Centers for Disease Control (CDC) issued a prediction: "Type 2 diabetes, once believed to affect only adults, is being increasingly diagnosed among young people. Unless American families change the way they eat and live, *1 in 3* children will eventually get diabetes."

- The front page of *USA Today,* November 3, 2008, reported on a study published in the medical journal *Pediatrics* that showed an alarming increase from 2002 to 2005 in the percentage of children on medications for chronic illnesses. The increase in children on medications for diabetes rose 103 percent; for asthma, 47 percent; for ADD and ADHD, 41 percent; and for high cholesterol, 15 percent. The study also showed a gender difference. The number of boys taking medications for diabetes increased by 39 percent, while the number of girls taking these medications skyrocketed 147 percent.

- Rather than "life expectancy," the WHO (World Health Organization) uses the more meaningful term "health expectancy" — the number of years one is expected to live in good health. The United States ranks twenty-fourth in health expectancy. I have heard many doctors at medical meetings say that this may be the first generation in history in which the children have a shorter "health span" (or health expectancy) than their parents.

- The number of preschool children who are receiving mood-altering drugs, either to perk them up or calm them down, has tripled.

- The number of Ritalin prescriptions for two- to four-year-olds has tripled.

- The number of prescriptions for mood-altering psychotropic medicines (SSRIs, like Prozac) for children younger than five years old has increased tenfold.

- Allergies serious enough to be debilitating and require drug treatment have increased an average of 5 percent per year.

- The Bogalusa Heart Study revealed that 60 percent of overweight five- to ten-year-olds already showed signs of cardiovascular disease. In July 2008 the American Academy of Pediatrics issued a historic recommendation that some children as young as eight years old be prescribed cholesterol-fighting drugs to prevent future heart problems, stating, "The advice is based on mounting evidence showing that damage leading to heart disease, the nation's leading killer, begins early in life." (My concern with this recommendation is that cholesterol is a vital structural component of brain tissue. When we tinker with the body's natural cholesterol-making mechanism, we run the risk of causing more NDD.)

- Obesity extreme enough to disable a child has increased 40 percent.

- GERD (gastroesophageal reflux disease) is now one of the most frequent diagnoses in children. Drugs previously reserved for heartburn in older folks are now frequently prescribed for children. Twenty years ago, GERD didn't even exist in the list of typical childhood diseases.

WHY SO MANY D'S?

The biggest D of the decade—ASD—or autism spectrum disorder, has reached epidemic proportions. Autism now affects one in 150 children. Nearly every day in our pediatric practice a parent asks, "Why are so many kids getting autism, and what can we do about it?" While there are many theories about what causes this neurological disorder, I believe that it is exacerbated by the polluted food that children eat and the polluted air that they breathe.

In the past year, an increasing number of studies have focused on the large number of schools throughout the United States that are located near polluted air. A 2008 study of 127,000 schools found that 20,000 of them are within half a mile of a major industrial plant. This is especially troubling because, as toxicologists have long known, a child's immature immune system makes him or her particularly vulnerable to the harmful effects of environmental pollutants, dubbed the "smokestack effect."

A BRAIN AND BODY OUT OF BALANCE

Once upon a time, the causes of ADHD and many mood, behavioral, and learning disorders were unknown. New insights into neurochemistry have shown that most of these Ds are due to neurochemical imbalances in the brain. In fact, psychiatrists often justify the use of drugs by telling patients that their Ds are due to a "chemical imbalance" that drugs will help correct. But balancing one bit of chemistry causes lots of imbalances in other bits. The typical child has the right balance of exciting and calming neurohormones. The child with ADHD, for example, is out of balance — too many exciting and not enough calming neurohormones. Why not balance the body and brain with food?

My Harvard Healthy Food Experience

Recently I was invited to a nutrition conference at Harvard Medical School to share the success stories of our LEAN Start Program (the health program we teach our patients, and the seven simple steps you will learn in this book). My presentation was near the end of the conference, and it followed talks given by professors of nutrition and experts in the field of nutritional biochemistry. Realizing that the audience was already overfed with statistics of the epidemic of Ds but underfed with real solutions to fixing the Ds, I decided to get real. So after my lecture I invited questions from the confused audience. "What about kids eating too much?" was the first question. "Just serve *real foods*. It's hard to overeat them," I answered. "Don't kids need a *low-fat* diet?" one audience member wondered. "No, they need a *right-fat* diet," I replied. "American families need an *oil change!*" I reminded them that mother's milk, the nutritional gold standard for optimal growth, is 40 to 50 percent fat. "Shouldn't kids be on a *low-carb* diet?" someone asked. "No, they should be on a *right-carb* diet," I corrected. To emphasize my point, I reminded this esteemed audience that the growing brain is 60 percent fat and that it utilizes carbs as the only source of fuel. "Shouldn't we have more nutrition education programs for parents?" someone suggested. "Yes, just tell them to serve *real foods*," I said. After the conference, a young medical student thanked me for simplifying the solution for the epidemic of Ds: *Eat real foods.*

NDD AFFECTS MIND AND BODY

While the effects of NDD are most noticeable in children's brains, nutritional deficit disorder also bothers growing bodies.

Mental Ds
ADD (attention deficit disorder)
ADHD (attention deficit/ hyperactivity disorder)
BPD (bipolar disorder)
DD (developmental delay)
Depression
LD (learning disability)
OCD (obsessive compulsive disorder)
ODD (oppositional defiant disorder)
SPD (sensory processing disorder)

Physical Ds
Allergic diseases
CVD (cardiovascular disease)
Diabetes
GERD (gastroesophageal reflux disease)
IBD (inflammatory bowel disease)
Infectious diseases (weak immune system)
Inflammatory diseases ("-itis" illnesses: e.g., dermatitis, colitis, bronchitis)
Vision deficiencies

Neither the food industry nor the government is going to cause the Ds to drop. Parents must be the change agents. They are at the top of the food supply chain: Farmers grow it, the food industry packages it, supermarkets stock it, and parents buy it.

PURE MOMS TO THE RESCUE

Years ago in my pediatric practice, I noticed that more and more mothers were feeding their children healthfully. Initially, I reacted like the typical nutritionally misinformed doctor and dubbed them health nuts. Later I called them "pure moms." As I finally began to get the message that food was medicine and that NDD was at the root of many of the Ds, I started using my medical practice as a nutritional laboratory. I decided to study what these moms did and how their children turned out, and to offer some nutritional tips of my own.

They served real food. After starting life with real food from Mom's body, these "pure kids" continued to get real food from Mom's kitchen. Instead of food from jars or cans, these children got real veggies prepared fresh, and cookies made from scratch. Yum! With a kid-friendly nibble tray full of nutritious "grow foods," they grazed their way through toddlerhood, eating when hungry, stopping when full.

They practiced the "we principle." They taught their children, "This is what *we* believe, this is how *we* dress, this is how *we* talk, and this is what *we* eat." Pure and simple! When their kids fussed for junk food, these motivated moms lovingly but uncompromisingly said, "We don't eat that in our house." They not only made food pure, they made food fun. Realizing that kids are more likely to eat the foods they grow, they planted gardens together. They called the produce "grow foods." Kids like that term. These moms seldom used the term "healthy," because some children equate healthy with icky.

They made feeding fun. They understood that they were bucking the trend and that their pure children would soon enter the polluted world, so they realized they had to serve quality food in a creative way. For example, they made fresh pizzas with funny faces. Eating was fun! They also went out of their way to help food taste better so that their children developed a taste for real food (see our recipes, chapter 12). Their children had normal sweet tooths (mother's milk is one of the sweetest of all foods), so they wanted their children to develop a taste for real sweetness from fruits. These kids learned, for example, that plain yogurt sweetened and colored with blueberries was a better grow food than yogurt diluted with fake colors and sweeteners.

They did "traffic-light" eating and shopping. These mothers regarded the supermarket as a giant nutritional classroom and taught their children how to have fun shopping. They played nutritional games when approaching the produce section, saying things like "Go pick out three reds, two blues, and four yellows," to teach their kids that the more colorful a food, the better a grow food it is likely to be. They taught them to shop the perimeter of the supermarket "because that's where the grow foods are." At my suggestion, they taught their children the concept of "traffic-light" eating: green-light, yellow-light, and red-light foods. Children loved the green-light foods ("eat them anytime and eat them as much as you want" foods). They learned that green-light foods helped them grow stronger and run faster. Yellow-light foods were "eat sometimes" treats. They learned there was an aisle in the supermarket that "we just don't go down," where the red-light foods were. These pure children learned very quickly that red-light foods kept them from growing strong and caused them to miss school and games and to have dry skin and less pretty hair and to just not feel well. (For more information about traffic-light eating, see page 77.)

They taught the three bad words. When their kids learned to read, these moms taught them how to read labels: "Look for good words on the label, like *whole grains.* Beware of the three bad words on the label: *high fructose corn syrup, hydrogenated,* and *anything with a number,*" or what they called the "yucky stuff."

They shared with pure families. Realizing that peer pressure influenced eating habits, these pure parents went out of their way to dine with other pure families so that their kids would understand that real foods are normally eaten in other houses too.

METABOLIC PROGRAMMING – A KEY TO ADULT HEALTH

Metabolic programming is a new and exciting field of research that relates early feeding experiences to later adult diseases. Studies have revealed that breastfed infants, compared with formula-fed infants, tend to have lower cholesterol as adults. The theory goes that, since breast milk contains cholesterol, and infant formula doesn't, adults who were breastfed are able to metabolize cholesterol better because these mechanisms were turned on early.

The term *imprinting* is sometimes preferred over metabolic programming because it suggests something that cannot be forgotten. Parents try to imprint many habits, such as their faith and values, on their children when they're young in the hope that even if their children should later deviate from these early habits, they will eventually return to them because they have been so

From one mother: "All my friends comment about how even-tempered and easygoing my children are. I know that temperaments are partially inherited, but I really do think that diet has a lot to do with behavior. When my kids get too much junk food, they become whiny and have extremely short attention spans. They even complain of headaches."

They prepared their kids for the real world. When these pure kids got out into the impure world of birthday parties, school lunches, and teen pizza pig-outs, of course they picked at the formerly forbidden foods, but the difference was, they didn't overdose, for two reasons: (1) Their tastes had been shaped toward only real foods, so fake foods tasted foreign to them; and (2) Their growing little guts had been programmed at the biochemical level to expect and digest only real food. (You will learn more about

deeply imprinted on them. Yet parents often forget about nutritional imprinting. One of the most heavily researched areas of nutritional imprinting is the link between early obesity (children who are overfed but malnourished) and later diabetes.

Metabolic programming researchers believe that during childhood, there is a window of nutritional opportunity to imprint lifelong nutritional habits that will program children at the cellular level to grow up to be healthy adults. I call this a "programming window." It seems that the genetic code of the cells "memorizes" feeding patterns and encodes them into lasting "this is the way we're supposed to behave" actions.

At this writing, metabolic, or nutritional, imprinting research is in its infancy. So, parents, let's use the science of common sense. Let your children's rapidly growing genetic codes memorize the effects of eating real foods. As a result, when your children become adults, they are more likely to enjoy good health.

"grow foods" in chapter 4.) Because of this real-food programming at the gut level, when fake food entered those preprogrammed little guts, some inner voice said, "Reject!" As a result, these kids learned at the gut level, "I eat well, I feel well; I eat badly, I get a case of yucky tummy."

Teachers noticed a difference. When other children were going to all their D doctors (ADD therapists, OCD therapists, allergic disease specialists, etc.), the pure kids who ate real food were simply doing real-kid activities — playing sports and games. Teachers noticed that these kids were *d*elightful to have in class. Not only were they healthier and did they miss less school, they were better focused, better behaved, and less moody.

I noticed a difference. These pure kids not only got sick less often, but when they did get the usual childhood infectious diseases, they healed more quickly. When these kids went to school, I saw them less often for the behavioral and learning Ds. When they got to be teens, I saw them less for the moody Ds of depression and anxiety disorders. When these pure children of pure parents became parents themselves, they fed their children real food simply because that's what their mothers did.

Wellness is less expensive. Initially some of the pure moms who were living on a tight budget worried that it might cost more to feed their children pure foods, but they realized that it actually costs less: With fewer Ds, there were fewer doctor bills and fewer missed days from work. Wellness is certainly less expensive than illness! Prevention is less expensive than treatment.

While primarily written for parents to prevent and reverse NDD in their children, this is really a book for people of all ages. NDD, like adult ADD, is a disorder we can have at any age, and the treatment is the same for all. My hope is that this book will be required reading for every childbirth class, for every applicant to day care, and for every parent at their child's school entry. I would like this book to be the first prescription from D doctors, either before or in addition to drugs, along with the advice, "Read this and do this first, and I'll see your child again in a month."

Parents, make a change. I guarantee you will notice a difference in your child's focus, behavior, and health. You will love the difference you see. My commitment to you: I am a show-me-the-science kind of doctor. Every nutritional statement in this book is scientifically correct. My hope for you is that you get a call from your child's teacher saying, "His behavior is so much better," and kudos from your doctor saying, "He's not sick as often as he used to be. Whatever you are doing, keep it up!" And that at some distant time you get a hug from your child saying, "Thanks, Mom and Dad, for giving me the gift of health."

2

You Are What You Eat: How Fake Food Causes NDD

As a pediatrician, I wonder how so many smart moms and dads, who truly love their children, can feed their family so much fake food. I believe it is because they don't really understand how junk food harms their children or appreciate how real food will help their children grow smarter, healthier, and happier. After you read this chapter, you will want to feed your family only real food.

My interest in how food acts in the body began when I noticed that the pure kids I talked about in chapter 1 didn't suffer from as many Ds as the junk-food eaters did. I imagined that if I could do a biopsy of the pure kids' gut linings and brain tissue, it would show that these tissues were healthier. I started reading biochemical journals to find out if the bodies of these pure kids might be different at the cellular and biochemical levels. There is plenty of information to support the axiom "you are what you eat," but it is found only in journals such as the *American Journal of Clinical Nutrition,* which don't get read and appreciated by parents or even by many doctors. By making these studies come alive, I want to motivate parents to change how and what they feed their families.

Feed a balanced brain and body. Optimal growth and development occur when a growing body is in biochemical balance. In fact, a good definition of health itself could be "the state in which biochemical balance exists in the body," a concept that has been appreciated in Eastern medicine for centuries. It is only recently that it has been shown scientifically. One reason we have so many Ds in our schools is that we have so many little bodies that are out of biochemical balance.

Until recently, I did not understand why intelligent parents weren't cleaning up their child's nutrition. They otherwise protected their children, guarding them from predators on the playground, screening movies in theaters, and modeling ethical and moral living at home. But they weren't carrying this protectiveness over to their children's growing brains and bodies. But I now realize that it's not that parents don't care; it's that *many parents just don't know the facts.* They are not convinced that fake food harms and real food helps growing brains and bodies. Read on and you will be committed to being a pure parent.

BRAIN FACTS YOU NEED TO KNOW

Think about how valuable your child's brain is. It enables your child to learn and to love; to laugh and to cry. More than any other organ, the brain is affected — for better or worse — by what your child eats. The brain deserves the best food. The good news is that while the brain can quickly deteriorate from NDD, it can also quickly rebound.

What to know. The brain grows faster in the first five years than at any other time in a child's life. The brain triples in volume by age two years and reaches 90 percent of its adult size by age five. By age six, a child has more connections (called *synapses*) than at any time in his or her life. After that, the brain selectively prunes unused or unneeded pathways.

What to do. Feed your child smart foods, not dumb foods, during this stage of rapid brain growth.

What to know. The brain is the most food-sensitive organ in the body, requiring a slow and steady supply of energy.

What to do. Feed the brain slow foods, not fast foods. (You will learn about slow-release carbs on page 43.)

What to know. The brain is 60 percent fat.

What to do. Children need a right-fat diet, not a low-fat diet.

What to know. The brains of growing children use more than 50 percent of the total energy they get from food for growth and function, much more than the 20 to 25 percent used by the adult brain.

What to do. Feed children enough real food to get real brain growth.

What to know. Pollutants and food additives are stored mostly in fat tissue, and the brain is mostly fat.

What to do. Feed children food free of additives and pesticides to limit storage of these chemicals in the brain.

What to know. The brain uses only carbs for fuel and, unlike other organs, the brain does not store sugar.

What to do. Feed your child the right carbs at the right times and encourage grazing for a steady supply of fuel.

What to know. Because the brain is so vulnerable to the effects of environmental toxins and junk food, nature has provided a protective layer of cells strategically located between the blood vessels and brain tissue, called the *blood/brain barrier* (BBB). But the BBB is underdeveloped in young children.

What to do. The younger your children, the more pure food they need. Their brains are not designed to run on fake food.

WHAT GOES ON IN THAT GROWING BRAIN?

Since the brain is the control center of the body, when the brain is affected, so is the entire body. Let's go inside your child's brain, the organ most affected by NDD.

Take a trip inside the brain cell. Your child grows because individual cells grow and multiply. Health 101 states that the body is only as healthy as each cell in it. Magnify that message for *growing* bodies and brains, when cells are dividing into new cells millions of times a minute. The contents of a brain cell are held together by the cell membrane, a flexible bag magnificently designed to protect all the structures inside the cell, such as where the energy is produced and the genes replicate themselves, and where all the biochemical action occurs. The cell membrane communicates with tiny branches of the bloodstream that flow next to it. Nutrients from the foods we eat seep out of a tiny capillary through the cell membrane and into the cell to feed the genes and the microscopic energy machines called *mitochondria.*

A malnourished membrane is the root of NDD. The most important thing you need to know about the cell membrane is that it's selective. This biochemical perk, which is called *permeability,* lets in just the nutrients that the membrane needs and keeps out the harmful stuff it doesn't need. But a malnourished cell membrane becomes stiff and stubborn and doesn't let the good nutrients in and keep the bad stuff out. And when cell membranes don't behave properly, the whole body misbehaves.

It is important to understand these two facts about cell membranes:

- They are composed mostly of fat.

- Built into the surface of these membranes are millions of microscopic "parking places," biochemically known as *receptor sites*. The membrane can tell whether or not a nutrient or a chemical in the blood is good or bad for the cell by whether or not the nutrient fits into these receptor sites.

One way to look at these receptor sites in the cerebral communication system is as locks and keys. The receptor sites are the locks, and chemical messengers, called *neurotransmitters,* are the keys. Real food feeds these messengers; fake food doesn't. Fit the right keys into the right locks and you have good health. Jam the wrong keys into these locks and you have illness. Remember this lock-and-key analogy about the cell membrane because it is vitally important to understanding how real food makes cells grow healthy and prevents NDD, and fake food causes NDD.

The neurotransmitters, the "keys," are made mostly of proteins, while the receptors, the "locks," are made mostly of omega fats. Yet the standard American diet (SAD), especially breakfast, is sadly deficient in these two nutrients.

One day I was counseling parents on how to help their child learn and behave better at school. After "checking the oils" in this child's diet, I felt like saying, "Your child's brain is full of molecular misfits."

Suppose you are a cell builder and you want to make the healthiest cell membrane. Naturally, you choose the best building materials, and that's what the body in its wisdom wants to do. Since the number one structural component of cell membranes is fat, the *healthier the fats, the healthier the cell membrane, and the healthier the child.* It's really that simple!

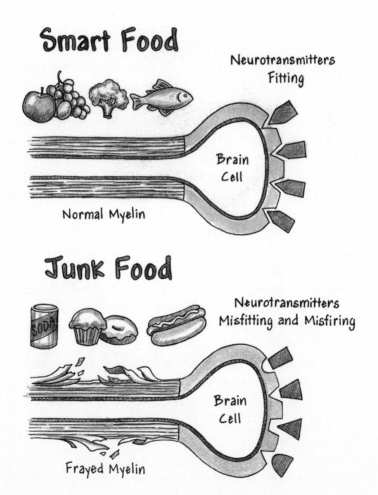

Since brain tissue is mostly fat, and the brain needs so much sugar for fuel, let's move on to the right-fat and right-sugar diet for growing brains.

NEW RX FOR THE D'S: GO FISH!

Suppose your child is diagnosed with one of the Ds, such as ADHD, OCD (obsessive compulsive disorder), or BPD (bipolar disorder), and you are a show-me-the-science parent. You find the top D-doctor in your city, and in you go for a consultation. After interviewing you and your child, top D-doc hands you a prescription for salmon or a bottle of fish oil. Don't laugh! There is more research attesting to the safety and efficacy of omega 3s for the Ds of the brain than there is for psychotropic medications. There are over twelve thousand medical journal articles on the health benefits of omega 3s, especially for growing healthy brains and hearts.

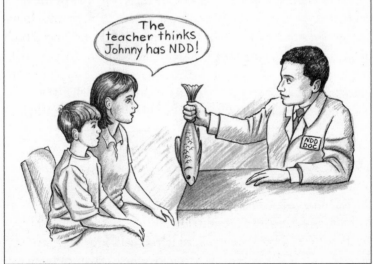

A TALE OF TWO BRAIN FATS

Let's follow two types of fats into the cell membrane to see how the good fats, omegas, produce wellness, and the bad fats produce illness. Your child eats a fillet of wild salmon, which happens to be the top brain food and to have the healthiest fats. These fats are called *essential fats* because the brain can't function without them, and the body can't live without them. The body can't manufacture them, however, so you have to eat them. The wild salmon contains two types of smart fats, omega 3s and omega 6s, in just about equal amounts. It just so happens that the cell membrane needs both of these. The omega 3s and the omega 6s are friends. They play together and they build together. When they play nicely together and one doesn't try to overpower the other, they build healthy cell membranes together.

By a beautiful design of nature, within the cell membrane are built-in biochemicals called *enzymes* that place these two fats together to build a structurally sound membrane with just the right configuration of locks for the nutrients, the keys, to fit into. In order for these locks to have the right configuration, they need both of these fats. And there are builder enzymes that act like bricklayers, piling up one omega 3, then one omega 6, then another omega 3, and then another omega 6. As long as the 3s and 6s come into the bloodstream in just the right amounts, the structure of the cell is strong.

What happens when smart brains get a dumb oil change? Suppose that Mom is shopping with her child and they go right past the seafood counter into the aisle full of chips and other foods with too much of the omega-6 oils, and the child starts gobbling up these fake foods. Omega 3s, which actually are the favorite fat of the brain, spoil easily or turn rancid (which is why unfresh fish

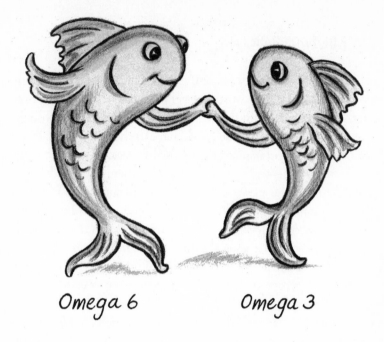

Omega 6   Omega 3

stinks). Omega 6s, however, can sit on the shelf for a longer time and not spoil. (If you're a fake-food maker, you would, therefore, use mostly omega 6s.) The child starts eating more fake food (which is less costly because it doesn't spoil). As a result, there are many more omega 6s in the bloodstream than there are omega 3s, and both of these fats arrive at the brain cell membrane. The builder enzymes on the brain cell say, "Oh my gosh, I've got so many omega 6s to manage that I have no time left over to manage the 3s." So the 6s, like neighborhood bullies, take over, and the 3s are left out of the cell membrane building.

Three things happen as a result:

- *In the wall of the cell membrane, the locks and the keys don't fit, so the membrane becomes less selective.* It may not let enough of the right nutrients in or keep the toxins out.

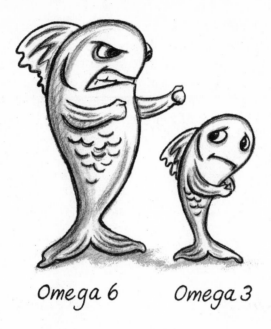

Omega 6   Omega 3

When the brain cell membrane is less healthy, the cell is less healthy and the whole brain is less healthy.

- *The nerves don't fire as fast.* Extending from each brain cell is a long filament like a tentacle on an octopus. This is how brain cells communicate with one another and how nerve messages travel, store memories, and communicate with the rest of the body, such as in telling the child to quickly raise her hand when she knows the answer to a teacher's question in class.

- *The omegas don't make as much myelin.* A substance called *myelin* makes nerves fire faster and communicate better. Myelin, like insulation on electrical wire, is composed mostly of fat, mainly omega-3 fats. Just like the electrical wiring in

your home, the better the insulation, the safer and more efficiently the electrical currents travel. However, if the omega
6s have stolen the builder enzymes from the omega 3s, the
omegas make less myelin. The myelin doesn't get enough 3s,
so it becomes like frayed insulation on electrical wires. The
child's brain gets fuzzy, forgetful, and quirky because the cell
membrane and the myelin are quirky.

The correct ratio of omega 3s to omega 6s varies throughout the
cell membranes of the body. In the cell membranes of the brain,
3s predominate because they are flexible fats, meaning they are

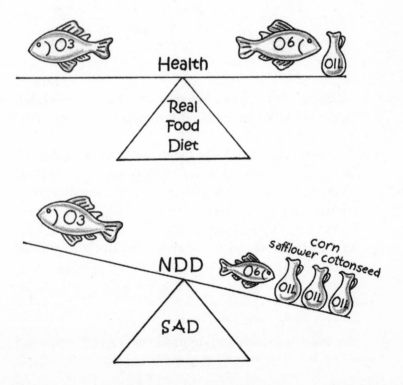

able to do many jobs and to fit in where they are needed. Because the brain has so many different jobs to do, it needs the most flexible fats to make the nerves work in many different ways. When the 3s and 6s are balanced, the child thinks and acts in balance. When the 3s and 6s are out of balance, NDD results.

Think of the body in biochemical balance like a country in political balance: It has peacekeepers to promote the health and welfare of a society, and a military force to protect and fight problems when necessary. Each group is fed an appropriate funding. As long as each group operates wisely, the country is healthy. Suppose there is a military takeover and the military gets too strong and influential, making wars and even attacking the people it was supposed to protect. This country is out of balance.

The same thing happens in the body. Omega 6s feed the military; omega 3s feed the peacekeepers. Both are good fats. Yet, when the 6s get higher and the 3s get lower, the body shifts into military mode and attacks itself: airways wheeze (asthma); skin gets dry, itchy, and rough (eczema); the lining of the bowel gets attacked (inflammatory bowel disease and colitis); and we have an epidemic of "iBods," children and adults riddled with inflammatory or "-itis" diseases.

If your child eats predominantly packaged fats with too many omega 6s, her brain tissue is going to be stiff and less flexible. The standard American diet, or SAD, has more 6s than 3s (more than ten times as many). Omega 6s can act like a gang leader. If there are too many of them, they edge out the 3s, so the neighborhood, like the brain cell, becomes less healthy. What fats do you want in your child's brain cell membranes? An equal number of 3s and 6s, of course. (See the list of foods containing both on page 40.)

Omegas make "brain talk." The brain makes mood-mellowing hormones. These go by the cerebral word *neurotransmitters*. I call them molecular messengers because they talk to the brain and tell it how to feel, think, and act. Omegas, especially the 3s, provide the food that feeds these messengers and tells them how to behave. Brain cells talk to one another through a sender-and-receiver network. Healthy fats, like omega 3s, make the brain messengers travel faster and more efficiently. These good fats get into the receivers and tweak them so they are tuned in to receive messages. A deficiency of omega 3s can lead to behavioral and learning problem Ds, such as ADD or, increasingly, depression. As you will later learn, omega 3s are the safest antidepressants.

While there are many molecular messengers traveling through the brain as your child goes through a busy day of growing and learning, for simplicity let's put these neurotransmitters into two groups:

- *Happy hormones* (e.g., serotonin). When these are turned on and in balance, the child is calm and focused. When they are out of balance, the child is either too high and anxious or too low and depressed. (See the related section about serotonin and gut feelings, page 132.)

- *Smart hormones* (e.g., dopamine, norepinephrine). These perk up the brain, making the child more alert and eager to learn, store and retrieve memory lessons, and focus on the present activity, whether in the classroom or on the field.

Meg, a calmer and conditioner. If the "Meg" in omega 3 could talk, she would say, "I'm a calmer. I calm upset brains and hyperactive inflammatory systems." Nutrition deficit disorder leads to neurotransmitter deficit disorder, resulting in a child who can't focus, can't learn, and can't behave. And the biggest increase in prescription drugs in the last decade are in those that are touted to help children focus and be calm, and to relieve depression.

The pharmaceutical industry is capitalizing on "treating" what the food industry helps cause.

Dr. Bill's easy lesson. The nutritional logic of brain function goes something like this: ADD and other brain Ds are thought to be due to miswiring and misfiring of the neurotransmitter system. This neurotransmitter system is affected, for better or worse, by food. Therefore, food is very important in treating the Ds.

Infants are born with most of the brain cells they're going to have, but it's the connections between brain cells that account for brain growth. Simply put, *real food helps the developing brain make the right connections.*

Quirky kids need more omega 3s. Some children — I call them "quirky" kids — think, act, and learn differently because their brains are wired differently. Their brain cells are more vulnerable to the effects of junk food than those of other children, so they are more vulnerable to quirky learning, mood, and behavior issues — the Ds. Other children might not seem to be as bothered by junk food, but they are still bothered on the inside in that their cells, blood vessels, and all their other tissues are gradually being harmed. They are not really developing well. Some quirky kids have an edge because their smart mothers discover very early on that certain foods are not good for them, so they don't feed their children these foods. The children who "aren't bothered by junk food" are worse off. They'll potentially be sicker when they're older.

Ideally, the brains of growing children need a ratio of around 2:1 to 3:1 of omega 6s to 3s. How do nutritionists know what is the right ratio? They go back to what we find in nature. Human milk averages this ratio. The ratio of these fats in wild meats and wild fish is around 2:1. The average American diet is over 10:1. Does your child need an oil change?

The "hydrogenated bomb" hits the brain. What happens in these growing cell membranes when a child eats a really bad fat? Until recently, hydrogenated fat (aka trans fat) was added to almost all fast foods and snack foods. Let's call this fat "H" for harmful.

Unlike the 6s, which become bad fats only when you eat too many of them, there is nothing good to say about "H." He is the fakest, sickest, and dumbest of all fats. Not only does "H" provide absolutely no nutritional value for growing brains, but he actually can make them sick.

To understand how fake fats disturb brain function, remember that brain cells communicate with one another via a sender-and-receiver network. Think of the receivers on a brain cell membrane like parking spaces reserved only for the nutrients that the cell needs, such as omega-3 fats, which help configure the cell membrane parking spaces to fit the nutrient and neurotransmitter "cars" that are assigned to park in them. If the wrong fats jam the parking spots, brain function fails.

Here's how "H" acts like a bad boy in the brain and makes it sick with NDD. "H" gets into the parking spaces on the brain cell membranes and clogs them, so the good fats can't fit into the membranes where they're supposed to. As a result of this cellular mischief, the brain literally can't think straight. The brain gets dumber on the dumb fats instead of smarter on the smart fats.

Fats are designed to behave healthfully in the body. What makes some fat molecules, such as omega 3s, healthy is their flexibility. Healthy fats are able to twist and turn in just the way that each cell needs to use them. Because "H" attaches to the wiggly tails of the omega fats and makes them stiff, they pile up in the blood vessel like Pringles in a can and shut off blood flow instead of rolling freely through the bloodstream like popcorn in a popper. All the growing organs need nourishment to grow. Fake fats act the same way in your body as they do in the pantry: They stay stiff and sticky. In chapter 9, I'll show you how to play with your kids I Spy with My Little Eye to recognize "H" as the bad word on the label.

OMEGA 3S MAKE YOUR CHILD'S IMMUNE SYSTEM SMARTER

Let's leave the brain for a minute and enter your child's immune system, which is intimately connected to the brain and similarly affected by food. The immune system is at the root of another epidemic of Ds: allergic diseases. We also have an epidemic of "iBods," a term that I coined for children who have "-itis" illnesses, such as asthmatic bronchitis, gastroenteritis, colitis, dermatitis, and even arthritis. (The biochemical term for iBods is *cytokines*.) Children are getting more of these "-itis" illnesses than ever before. Asthmatic bronchitis, in particular, has skyrocketed over the past decade. Again, the reason is food — junk food! (See page 46 for more about how poor eating causes iBods.) Real foods feed the immune system, so it behaves well in the brain and body. Fake food makes the immune system misbehave. It's as simple as that.

Children with many of the behavioral Ds, such as ADD and OCD, tend to be more allergic, and again, NDD is responsible. Omega 3s are not only the prime structural and functional components of the brain but also the building blocks of the immune system. Here's how I explain it to kids: "Feed the miniature soldiers inside your body good foods and they become strong soldiers that fight germs and keep you from getting sick. If you feed these soldiers junk food, they don't fight well for you. It stands to reason that allergic diseases, such as eczema and asthma, occur more commonly in kids with an NDD brain.

Over the past decade, the number of autoimmune diseases, especially rheumatoid arthritis and colitis, have been increasing at younger ages. In these "-itis" illnesses, the immune system gets its signals mixed up and attacks healthy tissues instead of foreign germs. Omega 3s help the immune system get the signals straight. Omega 3s are anti- "-itis" foods, acting like a twenty-four-hour circulating maintenance crew that circulates throughout your child's body and brain to help these tissues grow optimally.

OMEGA 3S HELP KEEP YOUR CHILD'S BODY AND BRAIN IN BIOCHEMICAL BALANCE

"Eat a balanced diet" was Grandmother's greatest nutritional pearl. Because we don't understand the depth of this wise saying, we tend to dismiss it, but Grandmother could not have been more nutritionally correct. Balance is what health is all about. A child with NDD is a child whose brain and body are out of biochemical balance. These children are running around (or more frequently sitting around) with their bodies and brains out of biochemical balance. Let's go inside the child's body to understand how feeding your child according to the seven simple steps in part 2 of the book will put your child's body back in biochemical balance.

Meet your child's NDD-preventing biochemical messengers. Your child's thinking brain and growing body are normally a biochemical soup of circulating molecular-messenger hormones that act like miniature computers regulating bodily functions. (The biochemical terms for these are *prostaglandins* or *eicosanoids.*) These hormones act like molecular switches that balance bodily functions: stop/go, on/off, up/down, open/close, sticky/smooth. Like an airplane on autopilot that adjusts the controls to keep itself balanced to go up or down, these molecular switches regulate body and brain functions, turning these systems up or down when needed.

For simplicity's sake, let's call the eicosanoids ECs. ECs are the body's balancing act. They are the on/off switches of the body's chemistry. Some ECs open up or widen airways and blood vessels, others narrow or constrict them. For example, when the ECs called *leukotrienes* are out of balance, they constrict the airways and cause them to go into spasm or cause an asthmatic attack. Medicines called *leukotrienes inhibitors* are among the newest classes of asthma-control medications.

The body always has to be on "red alert." Blood vessels sometimes have to widen or dilate to allow more blood to get to an organ that needs it, say to the muscles while you are running a race. But the body also needs ECs to narrow some vessels, allowing more blood to be shunted to needier organs. The body needs ECs to cause the blood to clot when you cut your finger but also to enable the blood to remain thin and flow freely through the blood vessels. We need ECs to turn on our army of internal infection fighters to heal an infection and seal a wound, and we need them to turn our army off so it doesn't overfight and wear out the tissue. An imbalance of ECs is one of the causes of the epidemic of iBod illnesses at all ages.

ECs are particularly sensitive to the foods that feed them. Fake foods throw them out of balance; real foods keep them in balance. For example, the right balance of healthy fats (more omega 3s and fewer processed oils, especially hydrogenated oils) has the greatest influence on the balance of these molecular messengers. If a child eats more fake food and less real food, blood flow is turned down to the body and brain, airways constrict, so the child can't get enough air, wounds do not heal as quickly, and the immune system maintenance crew gets out of whack. On the other hand, when a child eats more real foods, especially the healthy fats in seafood, the body's molecular messengers are turned up: Brain traffic flows more efficiently, blood flows through all the tissues better, and the immune system stays in balance.

Omega 3s and omega 6s are the foods that most influence how these molecular messengers behave and stay in balance. Here's what science says about them: When a person eats too much of the omega-6 fats and not enough of the omega 3s (see list, page 40), the switches turn on for many of the Ds. On the contrary, a person who eats real foods, including a balance of omega 3s and 6s, and basically eats according to the seven steps you will learn throughout the rest of this book, tends to have more of these molecular messengers turn off the Ds.

One day I was at a water park with a group of kids and noticed them having fun on a Slip 'N Slide. It struck me then that the blood vessels throughout a child's body are like a Slip 'N Slide. If you put real food into the child's body, that real food, besides keeping the on/off switches in balance, also keeps the lining of the arteries smooth like Teflon, instead of rough like Velcro from eating junk food. In a nutshell, eating real food keeps the sticky stuff out of your arteries so the blood flows more freely and nourishes growing brains and bodies better.

Science Says: Kids Need More Omega 3s

There are two approaches to understanding brain food. One is common sense, which goes like this: The brain is 60 percent fat, and therefore it needs healthy fats. Then there is science. Here's where the smart fats/smart brain growth connection really shines. Let's see what science says about 3s and 6s and the right balance for growing children:

- Breast milk is the gold standard for growing infants, averaging 2:1 to 3:1 6s to 3s, depending on the mother's diet.

- Cultures such as Asian and some Mediterranean that eat more omega 3s and fewer omega 6s and more closely approach the 2:1 to 3:1 ratio of 6s to 3s (unlike the 10:1 ratio of the SAD) have a much lower incidence of nearly all the Ds.

- Researchers have found that ADHD children tend to have a higher ratio of omega 6s to omega 3s in their diet. Also, low levels of omega 3s in the blood of children studied were associated with more of the Ds, such as ADHD, OCD, and CDs (conduct disorders).

- Some children with ADHD were found to have low levels of the most brainy omega 3, DHA (docosahexaenoic acid).

- A study at Purdue University showed that children with balanced blood levels of omega fats tended to suffer fewer IDs (infectious diseases).

- Experimental animals whose diets were deficient in omega-3 fats were found to have smaller brains.

- A study of the brains of experimental animals who were given omega-3 supplements showed an increase in the number of dopamine receptors on their brain cells.

- Studies have shown that schoolchildren with the brain Ds, such as ADD, OCD, and depression, improved with omega-3 supplements. In 2005 the journal *Pediatrics* published some fascinating research called the Oxford-Durham Study. Researchers gave schoolchildren with learning problems daily doses of omega-3 supplements and noted marked improvement in their ability to learn. The results of this study were so convincing that teachers, unsuccessfully, lobbied to allow schools to dispense omega-3 supplements. (Certainly, it would lessen the Ritalin line at the school nurse's office.)

Here is a testimonial from the teacher of one of the students in the Oxford-Durham Study, an example of the handwriting of a six-year-old boy before and after omega-3 supplements.

**A Child's Handwriting Before
Omega-3 EPA/DHA Supplementation . . .**

to gau urstwet @gct
for Thewerms @n his
spaghetl@r Twet thput
up a really clevertrict

. . . and One Month After Supplementation:

To pay Mrs Twit back
for the worms in his
spagetti Mr Twit thought
up a really clever trick

GIVE YOUR CHILD AN OIL CHANGE

Change your children's oils, and you can change their lives. I believe that one of the most serious contributors to the epidemic of Ds and iBods is an imbalance of omega 6s and omega 3s. The good news is that this imbalance is easy to correct. If you feed your child more seafood and fresh food and fewer packaged foods, this real-food diet will naturally contain the right balance of omegas.

Clues That Your Child Needs an Oil Change

Here are some signs of omega-3 deficiency that I look for in my patients:

- poor school performance
- misbehaviors: impulsive, aggressive, angry
- mood swings: sad, angry outbursts, anxious
- vision problems: decreasing acuity, dry eyes
- skin: dry, flaky, scaly "chicken skin"
- allergies: asthma, hay fever
- "-itis" illnesses: dermatitis, bronchitis, colitis, arthritis
- a diet that contains mostly packaged foods

A Mother's Testimony After an Oil Change

My son had always been a happy, social, athletic boy, and a joy to be with ever since his adoption, at three years of age. Due to his prenatal exposure to heroin, methadone, and we are not sure what else, he was diagnosed with sensory integration syndrome. Simply stated, the neurons in his brain and body don't communicate properly. His difficulties started in the first grade: He had trouble concentrating, poor writing skills, and low grades at school. And his behavior at

THE OIL CHANGE YOUR CHILD NEEDS

Eat more of these oils	Eat less of these oils
These foods are low in omega 6s.	*These foods are high in omega 6s.*

• Best sources of omega 3s
   Fish oil supplements
   Seafood, fish oil
• Other sources of healthy
  omegas
   Flaxseeds, ground
   Flaxseed oil
   Nuts
   Olive oil
	Animal fats, such as meat
	Bakery goods
	French fries and most fried
	   fast foods
	Meats: feed-lot fed
	Corn oil
	Cottonseed oil
	Partially hydrogenated oils
	   (the worst). Don't eat foods
	   containing these oils.
	Safflower oil
	Soybean oil
	Sunflower oil

home was destroying all of us. He was lying, angry, and destructive. Any normal task would take numerous reminders and I felt like I was nagging constantly! He couldn't hold a thought, much less remember two or more consecutive tasks. He was failing second grade by the end of the first quarter, and his teacher simply didn't like him, due to his noncompliance and defiant behavior. His self-esteem had completely disappeared. I was being called in for meetings with the principal and the teacher weekly, and I was at my wits' end!

My son was diagnosed with moderate ADHD and oppositional defiant disorder, and an IEP had been developed for him, with special education and therapy services. He was scheduled to undergo more psychological testing and was already in therapy. I was told repeatedly by teachers, special education assessors, and all the other academic specialists that the only course of action that was proven to be successful was to put him on systemic ADHD medication. Just as I was about to give up and put him on the medication, my mother asked if I had looked into fish oil. Quite honestly, I thought it a bit odd, but I searched the Internet, found your Web site, and started him on fish oil the next day! Within two to three days, he was calmer, not "zoned out" or "spacey," just relaxed. He was still sharp, funny, and a bit sassy, but not disrespectful. Within a week, life at home was much less stressful, and he was getting along better with everyone. His sister even liked him, and there was laughter in my house again! Within two weeks, the evidence was also apparent in his schoolwork. His comprehension skills were above grade level, his writing was so legible, the teacher accused the substitute teacher of doing his work for him! We are now six weeks into our regimen of fish oil, positive affirmation, and visual learning, and our new life improves consistently. He is a happy and cooperative child. He now remembers and completes several consecutive tasks, and homework is not the ordeal it once was. We had spent thousands of dollars on tutoring, therapies, and various programs designed for learning-disabled children. Now he is at the top of his class and can rival his fifth-grade sister in several subjects.

This has been nothing short of our own personal miracle: You have given me my son back. Thank you, Dr. Sears!

HOW SUGAR FEEDS THE BRAIN: FOR BETTER OR FOR WORSE

I hope that I've convinced you to make an oil change in your family. Next, I'd like to address sugar. Guess which organ of the body needs the most sugar? The brain. But not just any sugar; it needs the *right* sugar. In fact, the brain can show quirky behavior when it doesn't get enough of the right sugars.

- Unlike other systems, such as the muscles, the brain does not store glucose. Therefore, your child needs a frequent supply. (See chapter 7, Raise a Grazer.)

- Unlike other organs that can break down fat and protein when there's not enough sugar to go around, the brain uses only glucose as its primary fuel.

- The brain is appropriately dubbed a "carbo hog," meaning that it utilizes more sugar than any other organ does. The growing brain of a child utilizes 50 percent of all the carbohydrates in the diet, much more than the 25 percent that an adult brain uses.

The brain likes "slow food," not fast food. Feed your child a *right*-sugar diet, not a low-sugar diet, and serve sugars that release energy slowly and steadily from gut to blood to brain.

A Tale of Two Carbs

Remember, the two buzzwords for carbo feeding the body and brain: *slow* and *steady*. You have already learned how a deficiency of healthy fats will bother the brain. In the typical SAD diet kids get a double whammy: too few smart fats and too many dumb sugars. Let's follow two carbs through the body and see how a good carb can perk up the brain and keep the body healthy and how a bad carb can bother the brain and make the body unhealthy.

Shaping sweet tastes. Suppose a child is hungry and eats a good-carb snack, such as an apple or one of the supersnacks listed on page 148. The first stop for the good carb is the taste buds. Because the good carb is partnered with friends, the sweetness is not as intense or artificial tasting, so the child's developing taste buds get used to the natural sweetness of fruit or a bit of honey

A CARB LESSON FOR YOUR CHILD: GOOD CARBS VS. BAD CARBS

Here's how I explain good carbs or "grow carbs" to my patients: "A good carb has two friends, fiber and protein. It never plays alone. [For children over seven, you can show them the "two friends" — fiber and protein — on the nutrition label on the package.] When the grow carb gets into your tummy, the two friends — fiber and protein — hold hands with the carb for a while so it doesn't rush into your brain too fast. As a result, you get a *slow* and *steady* release of the good carb for energy.

"A bad carb, however, has no friends. It plays alone. When it gets into your tummy, it rushes really fast into your brain and makes you hyper. And it gets used up really fast, so you get 'fuzzy' and hungry really soon. Which friend do you want to play with, the good carb or the bad carb?"

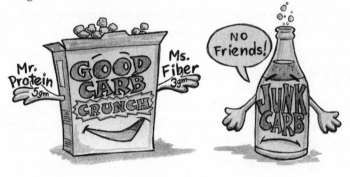

mixed with plain yogurt. Even the sweet taste of sugar (such as a teaspoon of sugar or honey added to a cup of oatmeal) is blunted a bit by its three friends — fiber, fat, and protein. With a bad carb, such as a corn syrup–sweetened beverage, the child's taste buds for sweetness are overwhelmed. If a child habitually drinks this bad carb, this is what he will associate with the normal taste and level of sweetness. Children whose tastes were shaped toward the sweetness that's found in nature, on the other hand, often find artificial sweeteners distasteful.

Also, because good carbs (such as an apple or a healthy crunchy snack) require a lot of chewing, more saliva is released. Saliva is the body's own health juice and digestive aid. It also accompanies the good carb and coats the stomach and intestines, so the good carb is associated with a good gut feeling. The bad carb, on the other hand, rushes through the mouth too fast and doesn't take much saliva with it.

In addition, the act of chewing on a crunchy carb helps a child be satisfied longer and curbs the urge to overeat.

Shaping good gut feelings. Next stop, the tummy. Because the good carb is partnered with the two friends fiber and protein, it stays in the stomach longer and is more filling and satisfying. Add a third friend, such as the healthy fat in peanut butter, and it stays in the stomach even longer and is even more satisfying. But the bad carb, because it has no friends, doesn't stay in the stomach very long and rushes right into the bloodstream, leaving the child hungry sooner.

The sugar rush hour. During the hour after eating, the sugar enters the bloodstream. The good (slow-release) carb seeps slowly into the bloodstream, while the bad (fast-release) carb rushes in too fast. And here's where the mischief of biochemical imbalance occurs. The level of carbs in the bloodstream sends a signal to its escort, the master hormone insulin, saying, "Escort me into places in the body that need me as fuel." Insulin comes alongside the good carb and ushers it into the cells of the body in just the right amount that the cells need. When the sugar rush of the bad carb hits the bloodstream, it commands lots of insulin to rush into the bloodstream. Now you have an excess of insulin and sugar traveling around the bloodstream, more than the body needs.

Insulin insults. The mischief begins at the cellular level. On each cell in the body are millions of microscopic "doors," called receptor sites. Insulin is like a doorman that ushers the glucose through these doors and into the cell. But when too many molecules of sugar hit these cells all at once, the cells need to protect themselves, and they close some of their doors to resist being overwhelmed by too much sugar. If this happens during many meals over many years, some of the doors on the cells stay closed, meaning they resist the ability of insulin to usher glucose through these doors — a condition called *insulin resistance,* or type 2 diabetes, the type that is causing the current epidemic and at younger ages. Besides all those Ds of the brain, the epidemic of diabetes is the most serious NDD affecting the body.

Junk sugars can make you sick. Excess sugar makes the child sick by depressing the immune system, mainly by weakening the ability of white blood cells, the body's internal germ-fighting army, to fight. Because good carbs are released slowly into the bloodstream, the body burns these carbs as needed. Bad carbs, on the other hand, rush into the bloodstream faster than the body can burn them. This high blood sugar depresses immunity.

Junk sugars can make you fat. The body doesn't like to waste food. All that excess sugar traveling around the bloodstream has to be stored somewhere. You guessed it — it gets stored right in those love handles around the middle. The belly becomes the storehouse for excess carbs. In my office I get a clue to a child's diet not only by measuring the blood sugar but by looking at the belly fat. In fact, in our medical practice we use waist size and excess abdominal fat as a more meaningful measurement than scale weight when it comes to weight control. We call it "waist" management rather than weight management.

This scene took place in my pediatric office: Eleven-year-old Melissa sat with her arms folded, obviously upset that her mother had dragged her into the doctor's office. Mother immediately jumped into the "something's wrong with my daughter, please fix it" mode. Meanwhile, Melissa gave her mother a look that conveyed, "Back off, Mom!" Mom got the message, and Melissa and I began a doctor-patient dialogue.

"Melissa, what activity do you like best?" was my icebreaker.

"Soccer," she quickly volunteered.

"Melissa, if you had one wish about soccer, what would it be?" I asked.

"I would like to run faster and not get out of breath so fast."

(Meanwhile, Mom was making gestures as if thinking, "Why doesn't he start talking about her being overweight?")

"So, Melissa, you'd like to run faster and breathe better. How about we talk about Dr. Bill's run-faster, breathe-easier 'program'?"

Melissa nodded in wide-eyed approval.

"Melissa, your body is full of iBods," I said. That surprised her.

"Sounds like iPods," she countered.

I explained. "iBods are millions of tiny particles that travel through the rivers of your blood and stick to your joints, which is one reason it hurts to run (arthritis). This iBod stuff also sticks to the inside of your arteries, so you don't get enough blood flow and nourishment to your tissues. That's why you get tired when you run. It also sticks to your airways, making it difficult to breathe or run (allergic bronchitis). And Melissa, notice your flaky, itchy skin (dermatitis). That's those iBods again."

"Where do these iBods come from?" she inquired.

"They start in junk food, especially junk carbs, and then settle around your waist. That extra flab is an iBod factory."

(Meanwhile, Melissa's mother finally got where I was going with this iBod stuff.)

"So we're going to close the iBod factory by trimming a lot of that extra fat around your middle. Our goal is to go down two jeans sizes in the next six months."

"Then you'll see Melissa and weigh her each month?" her mother persisted.

I corrected her: "Waist size is the only measurement we'll do. It's more meaningful than weight."

I gave Melissa a goal of dropping two inches off her waist size and being able to fit into smaller jeans over the next year. Three months later, Melissa was a happier, healthier preteen. She had dropped five pounds and, more important, three inches off her waist size. She proudly volunteered, "My jeans don't fit anymore, I have to get new ones!"

To most modestly overweight children and teens I give a "no-gain goal." If they stay the same weight and waist size over the next couple of years, because they're growing so fast, that is equivalent to an actual weight and fat loss. Through the natural "leaning-out" process, they gradually grow into their optimal weight and waist size.

(For a complete weight management program for families, see www.AskDrSears.com/LeanStartProgram.)

Junk sugars can make the brain misbehave. Not only is the body out of chemical balance, but so is the brain. When excess insulin causes tissues to use up the excess carbs too fast, the brain crashes. (Remember, unlike other tissues of the body, the brain doesn't store sugar, so it runs out of fuel more quickly.) While a steady supply of good carbs gives steady moods, junky carbs give junky moods, junky behavior, and junky learning — and the child gets labeled with more Ds, such as ADD, OCD, learning disabilities, and depression. Even some preschool children are getting labeled with bipolar disorder, meaning they fluctuate from very hyper to very depressed. There is a correlation between how children think and act and how they eat. Remember, the brain is not designed to run on unreal food.

Junk carbs stress the brain. Picture what's going on in the body of a child who has eaten a junky breakfast. While he is trying to sit still at a desk in a classroom and pay attention to what the teacher is teaching, the ups and downs of his blood sugar prevent his brain from learning, and the ups and downs of stress hormones keep his body and mind from behaving. So he tunes out the teacher and gets labeled with ADD, or he disobeys the teacher and gets labeled "oppositional defiant." The problem is that these Ds sprang from all the biochemical disturbances in his blood and brain.

Supersensitive children self-medicate. The sugar story gets even more sour. The brain, which has a lot of built-in protective mechanisms, senses something unsettling is going on, so it sends out signals to get the brain and body back into biochemical balance. The brain then talks to its helpers, the adrenal glands, the body's second command center, and says, "I need help up here. I ran out of fuel. Send me some sugar, fast!" So the child begins, in effect, to self-medicate. First, the adrenals pour out the stress hormones to draw stored sugar out of the reserve bank account in the liver. But these stress hormones also amp up the child's already unsettled biochemistry and result in unsettled behavior.

The brain then says, "I need more 'medicine' to treat the side effects of the stress hormones." The next prescription is "Move!" The brain knows that movement stimulates neurochemicals that mellow the mind, so the child fidgets with his hands and fingers, pumps his legs, and squirms his whole body. Meanwhile, the teacher shrugs off these self-medicating behaviors. "Oh, it's just his ADHD!" For many ADHD children, hyperactivity is their way of compensating for a brain out of balance.

Finally, the lunch bell rings, and now the child with NDD can grab more "medicine." He wolfs down more junk carbs, because carbs release the mind-mellowing neurotransmitter serotonin. In effect he gets a fix, and in reality he is functioning like an addict — a sugar addict.

Here's how addictions work. The brain is a creature of habit. Even though the brain is experiencing biochemical disturbances and ups and downs of mood and behavior, after a while the brain interprets these feelings as normal and eventually starts craving the feelings. The sugar-addicted child becomes a junk-carb craver and develops another D — dependency. The longer your child has been eating junk food, the longer it may take to wean him or her off it.

Quirky Kids Are More Sugar-Sensitive

Many children with the Ds, such as ADD, don't really have disorders, but they do have differences. They think, act, and learn differently. So they not only need a different style of parenting and teaching, they need a much healthier diet. Instead of labeling a child with ADD, I often use the term *quirky*. Quirky kids think outside the box. But given the right food and intervention, these kids can grow up to build better boxes.

The growing brains of some children are more sugar-sensitive than others. A fascinating study at the Yale University School of Medicine compared the effects of a high-sugar meal on the brain scans of children with ADHD with those of typical children, and they found amazing differences in how both of these groups of children reacted to the junk-sugar meal. Compared with typical children, the sugar-loaded children with ADD/ADHD showed:

- Lower scores on tests measuring their learning and attention.

- More fidgeting and physical movements three hours later when their blood sugar was low.

HOW FOOD TALKS TO THE GENES

An exciting new test is coming soon to your doctor's office! Suppose you have a new baby. At birth a sample of cord blood is analyzed for your child's "quirks," or genetic tendencies toward common diseases: cardiovascular disease, diabetes, cancer, Alzheimer's, and so on. Included in this test will be a printout of which foods increase this risk. Your doctor may then say, "Billy carries a genetic tendency toward insulin-resistant diabetes, so he absolutely should not drink soda."

This fast-growing field is called *nutrigenetics* (or *nutrigenomics*), and it focuses on how food "talks" to the genes. New discoveries show that if a certain genetic tendency is present, say, for diabetes, some foods "turn on" this gene, and the child eventually gets diabetes. Other foods can "turn off" the gene. While you can't change your child's genes, you can control the on/off switch by controlling how and what your child eats. Until this blood test becomes readily available, consider the sixteen superfoods listed on page 99 as foods that turn off the common disease genes, and the sixteen sick foods as ones that are likely to turn on these genes.

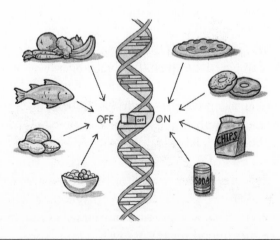

- Decreased ability to mobilize their sugar-raising hormones, epinephrine and norepinephrine, when their blood sugar got too low. This means that they were less able to self-regulate their blood sugar, so they were more vulnerable to "attacks" of low blood sugar.

In another study, when teens were given a high-sugar drink, the brains of kids with ADD/ADHD did not utilize the sugar as efficiently as the brains of typical kids did.

Children who are very sensitive to sugar may climb the walls after one soda; other children may appear unbothered after gulping twenty-four ounces. What is more worrisome? Surprisingly, the seemingly unbothered child is at greater risk for the Ds. If your child is obviously hypersensitive to sugary drinks, you probably just don't have them in your home. But for the apparently unbothered child, it's easy to get lax in your food choices. This child eats more junk food when he is young and pays the price with more Ds when he is older. Fake-food eaters may feel fine now but get sicker later.

The bottom line is, these kids need to graze on good carbs. (See chapter 7, Raise a Grazer.)

HOW FOOD ADDITIVES AFFECT CHILDREN'S LEARNING, MOOD, AND BEHAVIOR

Now that you have learned how the wrong fats and unreal sugars cause NDD, you will learn about the third cause: artificial food additives. There's a lot of chemical stuff added to food to make it more "tasty" and "colorful" and to "preserve it." These additives add nothing but more Ds, particularly in supersensitive children. And since toxins are stored mainly in fatty tissue and the brain is 60 percent fat, it stands to reason that the brain will be most bothered by chemical additives. Fake foods are a triple whammy to the brain: They are too low in brain-building fats, too high in brain-disturbing sugars, and more likely to contain additives, which further throw the body and brain out of biochemical balance. Here's what you should know about those chemical-sounding "bad words" in the fine print on the package label.

Aren't Food Additives Tested and Approved by the FDA?

Have you read the newspaper lately? Some drugs that the FDA approved as safe, such as some anti-inflammatories and mood-altering medicines, are proving to be unsafe. If we can't trust the FDA with safety advice for drugs, should we trust it when it comes to food? Even though health experts knew about the dangers of hydrogenated, or trans, fats to all the organs of the body, it remained in our food supply for decades. It took the FDA twenty years after the dangers were revealed to finally speak out, in 2006. But rather than ban hydrogenated fats entirely, they simply mandated that food companies reveal the presence of trans fats on the packaging (see page 32). Don't expect the FDA to protect children from chemical additives. Parents must protect their kids.

What's supposedly safe for adults may not be safe for children. Studies on food additives are done on experimental animals, usually rats, or on adults representing the "average human." The reasoning goes like this: If you give enough rats a certain chemical and the rats seem okay, then it must be okay for kids. The problem is that a child's brain and body chemistry aren't like either a rat's or an adult's. Young children are rapidly growing, and their tissues and dividing cells are much more vulnerable to the effects of chemicals. Strike #1!

Children have more body fat. Children have a higher percentage of body fat than adults do. Many chemical additives are stored in fat, so children can have proportionately more harmful chemicals stored in their bodies and brains. Also, proportionate to their body weight, children tend to eat more food than adults because they are growing and more active. More food, more additives eaten, more chemicals stored. Strike #2!

Chemical additives are not tested for long enough periods of time. The FDA gives a bunch of rats chemicals for a few months and sees if they're okay. If the rats pass the test, they then give it to humans (usually adult volunteers) for a short period of time, often twelve weeks. If the humans don't get sick, the FDA says it's safe. The problem is, these chemicals are eaten for years and years and stored in the body for years and years, not just for weeks or months. Strike #3! These chemicals should be *out* of a child's body.

The biochemically correct term for these chemical additives is *neurotoxins* (meaning, "poisonous to the nervous system"). Can you imagine how a few neurotoxins eaten several times a day for twenty years, a few brain cells lost each day, and a few mis-wired nerves can add up? There are no animal studies that could ever prove these additives safe. So, it's back to the science of common sense. We have an epidemic of Ds, none of these additives have ever been proven safe for children, and many have been shown to be neurotoxic in experimental animals. The conclusion? *They are not safe for your growing child!* This is especially true for children with quirky brain wiring. I have spent a lot of time researching food additives and have concluded that I will not allow them in my own family's kitchen or in the mouths, bodies, and brains of the children I love, and I urge you to do the same. (See the list of neurotoxins on page 59, and cut them from your family's diet.)

You may say, "They don't seem to bother her!" My answer: How do you know? Because of the body's marvelous reserve of blood vessels and brain tissue, it may take years to find out that your child has been losing brain cells along the way. One day I was discussing the effect of junk food on the brain with neurologist Dr. Vince Fortanasce, author of *The Anti-Alzheimer's Prescription.* I suggested, "Vince, I believe Alzheimer's begins in childhood." Dr. Vince replied, "You know, Bill, you're absolutely right!"

From one mother: *"I'm a schoolteacher. Children go out to play after a calm morning, and some of them always come back hyper. Without fail, when I ask the hyper ones what they have eaten, it's always foods with artificial flavors or colors in them."*

Kids are more sensitive to additives than adults are. A child's growing brain is more vulnerable to the neurotoxic effects of chemical food additives. The protective blood/brain barrier (see page 21) is not fully developed until late in childhood, so at a stage when the brain is growing most rapidly, it is at its most vulnerable. We could call this the *leaky blood/brain barrier* of early childhood. There is a critical period from birth to around ten years of age when the brain is most vulnerable to the effects of junk food, especially in some areas of the brain, such as the hypothalamus, the brain center that is involved in chemical balance in the body. It's interesting that the label of behavioral and learning Ds is applied most often during this stage of development.

Then there are problems at the pump. Within the brain cell membrane are microscopic pumps that let the right amounts of the right chemicals into the brain tissue to help it grow and function, and also keep the bad chemicals out. Neurotoxic chemicals can damage the pumps in the brain cell membranes, especially in growing brains.

SCIENCE SAYS: IF ANIMALS GET SICK ON IT, WHY FEED IT TO KIDS?

Nutrition scientists have long known that feeding young animals junk food results in sick grown-up animals. Here's what the science says:

- High doses of MSG fed to pregnant experimental animals can damage the brains of their babies.
- Young animals fed flavor enhancers such as MSG showed changes in brain cell development and grew up to become obese and have autism-like symptoms.
- Young animals fed a junk-fat diet grew up to show abnormalities in cholesterol metabolism.
- Young animals fed a junk-carb diet grew up to show abnormalities in the insulin receptor sites on their cell membranes and developed type 2 diabetes.

Parents, I hope you get the message: Feed young kids junk food and you get older kids with junk health.

Neuroscientists are concerned about the cumulative effect of these bad chemicals. They worry that low doses of chemical additives eaten over long periods of time can accumulate to toxic levels. While these neurotoxic effects are concerning at all ages, they are especially worrisome in growing brains and bodies.

Neurosurgeon Russell Blaylock, author of *Excitotoxins: The Taste That Kills,* estimates that the developing infant's and child's brain is *four times more vulnerable* to the damaging effects of neurotoxins than the adult brain is. Dr. Blaylock believes that certain food additives, especially MSG and aspartame, cross the blood/brain barrier and can cause the developing nerve fibers to

---

YOU ARE ALSO WHAT THE ANIMAL YOU EAT EATS

Consider this food chain. The healthy, range-fed animal gets trucked from farm to feed lot and is downgraded from real food to fake food. This fake food–fed animal grows fatty, weak tissues. Fake food yields fake muscles. Children eat these fatty, fake muscles, and then their own muscles get fat and weak. The fat profile of the milk from range-fed cows is much healthier than it is for milk from feed-lot cows, as is the nutritional profile of most wild versus farmed fish.

---

be miswired. One of the effects of this miswiring is what I call *premature pruning.* The brain grows like a tended garden, pruning connections that aren't needed and allowing more growth for the connections that are needed. Too many additives could lead to too much pruning.

Real food helps the developing brain make the right connections. What diet should your child be on? The Real Food Diet. It's as simple as that!

Flavor Enhancers Usually Mean Health Detractors

When you take the oily flavor of fats and the sweet taste of sugars out of foods, they don't taste as good. Food manufacturers chemically disguise this fact by adding flavor enhancers to fool the tongue. When foods are hyped as "low fat" or "low carb," it usually means they are high in chemical additives, the most notorious and most common of which is monosodium glutamate (MSG). Let's examine what science says about MSG. Here are my concerns and the reasons I've concluded that MSG should absolutely be banned from the brains of children:

MSG bothers the brain. MSG is made from an amino acid called glutamate. There are a lot of glutamate receptors throughout the brain. In fact, some anti-epileptic and mood-altering medicines actually work by interfering with these glutamate receptors. Dr. Russell Blaylock labels MSG an "excitotoxin" because that's how it works. MSG chemically excites, or rather, deceives, the receptors in the brain to believe, "This fake food sure tastes good."

MSG can make you fat. When you make an otherwise bland food taste better, kids want to eat more of it. Remember the potato chip ad campaign "Betcha can't eat just one"? You can't. MSG increases the craving for more of the chemical stuff. Obesity researchers gave experimental animals MSG in order to purposely make them fat. One of the ways it did so was by increasing blood levels of insulin, the fat-storage hormone. So not only does MSG hype up brain cells, it can stimulate the cells of the pancreas to secrete more insulin. Certainly, kids with ADHD do not need to be chemically hyped up in any manner. Here is an interesting "home science project" for you and your child. Do an online search for the side effects of excitotoxins, such as MSG and aspartame, and make a list. Then go back online and make a list of the signs and symptoms of ADHD. Notice the similarity between the two columns.

"But MSG and aspartame are approved by the FDA, so they must be safe," you might argue. Not necessarily so. MSG especially was grandfathered into the GRAS (generally regarded as safe) category in the late fifties before research proving its safety could be done. The FDA has received more health complaints about MSG and aspartame than any other chemical additives. It's no surprise that studies have offered conflicting results. Those funded by the monosodium glutamate and aspartame makers "prove" its safety; independent studies demonstrate otherwise.

The FDA allowed the conclusion "When in doubt, leave it in," but you owe it to your children to take a safer approach — *When in doubt, leave it out.*

In what foods can you find MSG? Because MSG has gotten a deservedly bad rep, food packagers now use aliases such as "hydrolyzed vegetable protein," "natural flavorings," and "yeast extract." During the writing of this book I made a search and discovery trip around a grocery store. Here are some foods that listed MSG, or one of its aliases, among the ingredients. (I suspected that other products contained MSG, but it was disguised by names I didn't recognize — and I had thought I knew them all.)

- Many sauces, such as spaghetti sauces, list "natural flavors," whatever that means.
- Many sauces and ravioli, contain disodium phosphate.
- Canned soups are among the biggest offenders.
- Some teriyaki sauces contain "hydrolyzed soy protein."
- Many soy sauces contain sodium benzoate.

When eating out, be sure to grill the restaurant about whether they add MSG to anything you've ordered. To increase the chances that you will get an honest answer, tell them your child is allergic to MSG. (Actually, in my view you're telling the truth, since I believe that all children have subtle allergies to these preservatives; some just show it more than others.) For an update on how MSG is hidden in foods see www.truthinlabeling.org.

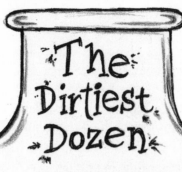

The Dirtiest Dozen

Avoid these chemical additives

as much as possible:

1. Partially hydrogenated oils
2. Aspartame (NutraSweet, Equal)
3. MSG (monosodium glutamate)
4. Hydrolyzed vegetable protein
5. BHA (butylated hydroxyanisole)
6. Acesulfame potassium
7. BHT (butylated hydroxytoluene)
8. Potassium bromate
9. Sodium nitrate and nitrite
10. Propyl gallate
11. Sodium benzoate
12. Artificial colors

Caution: May contain one or more

NDD-causing chemicals

ARTIFICIAL SWEETENERS – SOUR FOR CHILDREN

After thoroughly researching the most commonly used artificial sweeteners, aspartame (NutraSweet, Equal) and sucralose (Splenda), I concluded that I would not feed them to my children, and I discourage their use in my pediatric practice. In fact, I believe they are downright NDD-producing.

Aspartame – Bitter for Growing Brains

This artificial sweetener has been the most controversial for more than twenty years, and its safety still is not scientifically settled. In fact, aspartame has the dubious distinction of being a drug with one of the highest adverse-reaction reports to the FDA. Here are my concerns:

The science is skeptical. Many of the studies "proving" the safety of aspartame were funded by the manufacturers. Researchers have found that company-funded drug studies are four times more likely to report favorable outcomes than those conducted by independent investigators. In a 2008 scientific review of 160 studies of aspartame, 74 studies had aspartame industry–related funding, and 86 were independently funded. All of the industry-funded research supported aspartame's safety, and 92 percent of the independently funded research uncovered some kind of problem.

How the body breaks it down. Aspartame is a chemical compound composed of aspartic acid and phenylalanine. Phenylalanine is broken down into methanol, which is then broken down into formaldehyde. Yes, I did say *formaldehyde,* the embalming chemical. Yet aspartame supporters preach that this formaldehyde is rapidly metabolized into formic acid, which is then turned into water and carbon dioxide and rapidly excreted from the body. Supporters also say there is no reason for concern because the body has a built-in garbage disposal system to get rid of the breakdown products methanol and formaldehyde. However, a child's garbage disposal system is still maturing. Aspartame supporters also claim that the experimental animals that got sick on aspartame were fed much higher doses than humans would ever consume. Are we then to conclude that a little bit of aspartame may cause only a little bit of damage? My concern is about the cumulative effect of these little bits over a long period of time in growing brains.

Aspartame can make you fat. Aspartame is supposed to help you lose weight, but does it? Many researchers believe that artificial sweeteners can actually increase weight gain by increasing the body's craving for artificially sweetened food. The mere twelve calories fewer than a teaspoon of sugar isn't worth the chemical effect on a child's brain and body.

Aspartame bothers growing brains. The fact that a headache is the most commonly reported side effect of aspartame means it can't be good for the brain. Phenylalanine itself is a neurostimulant, just what a child with an already quirky neurochemistry doesn't need.

Sucralose (Splenda) — Also Sour for Children

Now that you understand why you must eliminate aspartame (NutraSweet, Equal) from your child's diet, let's add sucralose to the list of forbidden sweeteners.

Splenda is touted as "natural" because it's made from sugar. The manufacturer also claims that since the body does not digest or metabolize Splenda, it is a no-calorie sweetener. Wow! Made from sugar, tastes like sugar, but without the calories of sugar. Sounds like a dieter's dream. Read on.

What it really is. While Splenda may start out as sugar, here's where it becomes fake: Chlorine atoms are added to the sugar molecule, changing it into a chemical named 4,1',6' trichlorogalactosucrose. Scary, huh? Do you want to put chlorocarbons into your child's body?

How it behaves in the body. While the manufacturer claims that Splenda isn't absorbed into the body, if you read the fine print, you'll see that's really not true. The *Federal Register,* the official publication of the U.S. Food and Drug Administration, reveals that 20 to 30 percent of ingested Splenda *is* metabolized by humans. So the stuff really does get into the body, and no one is sure what it does when it gets there.

Tested mainly on animals, not children. Most of the tests on how the body metabolizes Splenda were performed on experimental animals (rats, rabbits, mice, and dogs), which metabolize biochemicals differently from humans. There have been no long-term studies done on the effects of Splenda on humans — on children or adults.

High Fructose Corn Syrup — Not So Sweet for Health

What about high fructose corn syrup as a substitute for sugar? Aren't they really the same? The scientific answer is, possibly, but we're not really sure. A few years ago I was on the TV show *The O'Reilly Factor.* After I made the case that hydrogenated fats may turn out to be the worst fake food in the history of the food industry, Bill O'Reilly asked me what I thought the next food on the hit list might be. I responded, "High fructose corn syrup."

I have four concerns about the safety of HFCS that convince me not to feed it to my own family.

1. HFCS is a molecular misfit. HFCS and table sugar appear to be very similar, since each is around half glucose and half fructose. HFCS is 55 percent fructose, 42 percent glucose, and 3 percent other sugars. Table sugar is 50 percent fructose and 50 percent glucose. How does the body handle the extra fructose in HFCS? We don't know. Table sugar is a disaccharide. This means that the fructose and glucose molecules are linked by a chemical bond. When sugar enters the intestines, this bond is broken down by the intestinal enzymes. Yet, with HFCS, the glucose and fructose molecules are not bonded to each other like the sugar molecules. They are more "free," since the intestinal enzymes are not needed to unbond the two sugars. While HFCS proponents claim that the body can't really tell the difference, we really don't know if this is true. Some research claims the extra fructose can cause molecular mischief in the liver, boosting blood levels of triglyceride fats and LDL (the heart-harming) cholesterol, while decreasing the HDL (the heart-healthy) cholesterol.

2. HFCS does not occur in nature. Since HFCS is produced in a factory rather than grown as a plant, like real table sugar, the body may not have developed mechanisms to metabolize it. Common sense tells us that if you put high doses of fake foods in a body that has not had millennia to adapt natural mechanisms to metabolize it, you pay a high health price. Since science can't agree on the safety of HFCS, I'll go with common sense.

3. HFCS is easier to overconsume. While studies are mixed, some obesity researchers believe that HFCS is a very low-satiety food: Because it's a fake sugar, it doesn't trigger hormones that naturally tell the body to stop eating or drinking.

MISSHAPING YOUNG TASTES

Besides the fact that artificial sweeteners have never being proven safe and are possibly harmful to a child's growing body, I am also concerned that they shape young tastes in the wrong direction. The three magic words in preventing NDD are *shaping young tastes* toward favoring real food. Artificial sweeteners sabotage this goal by shaping young tastes toward craving fake food. Putting these unproven chemicals into your child's body is not worth the few calories you may save. The safety of artificial sweeteners, especially for children, is still being argued among researchers; see www.AskDrSears.com updates for the newest information. Until then, concerning any fake food, my advice is *When in doubt, leave it out.*

---

4. HFCS is guilty by the company it keeps. While the safety of HFCS is likely to be argued in nutritional circles for the next decade and I don't believe it will ever be proven to be as harmful as trans fats, I put it on the "bad words" list for food labels because HFCS is guilty by association. It just so happens that the junkiest foods are the ones with the most HFCS. High fructose corn syrup is an easily identifiable target when teaching children how to recognize junk food. If you see HFCS on the label, the quality of all the other ingredients on the label is suspect.

A Tale of Two Chickens

Some parents might not appreciate the nutritional differences between fake food and real food. Consider the difference between Chicken McNuggets and nutritionally sound homemade chicken nuggets.

CHICKEN MCNUGGETS

Ingredients*
White boneless chicken, water, food starch–modified, salt, chicken flavor (autolyzed yeast extract, salt, wheat starch, natural flavoring [botanical source], safflower oil, dextrose, citric acid, rosemary), sodium phosphates, seasoning (canola oil, mono- and diglycerides, extractives of rosemary). Battered and breaded with: water, enriched flour (bleached wheat flour, niacin, reduced iron, thiamin mononitrate, riboflavin, folic acid), yellow corn flour, food starch–modified, salt, leavening (baking soda, sodium acid pyrophosphate, sodium aluminum phosphate, monocalcium phosphate, calcium lactate), spices, wheat starch, whey, corn starch. Prepared in vegetable oil ((may contain one of the following: Canola oil, corn oil, soybean oil, hydrogenated soybean oil with TBHQ and citric acid added to preserve freshness), dimethylpolysiloxane added as an antifoaming agent)

DR. PETER SEARS'S HEALTHY CHICKEN NUGGETS

Ingredients
Organic, hormone-free boneless skinless chicken breasts, sea salt, black pepper, ricotta cheese, omega-3-enriched egg, all-purpose flour, regular or whole wheat bread crumbs (See the recipe on page 191.)

---

*Accurate as of November 2008.

FOOD SENSITIVITIES: KEEP A FOOD-MOOD DIARY

To detect which foods cause which behaviors, keep a record like this one:

Food-Mood Diary

Quirky Behavior	Foods Recently Eaten

This is the same detection strategy parents use to detect food allergies. After a while, you will be able to correlate which foods contribute to which behaviors and get them out of your child's diet.

3

Ten Steps to Prepare Your Family for the Change

Before you make over your kitchen, you first have to make over your mind. Change is not easy for most families. In this chapter, you will learn ways to change your own mind and habits in preparation for changing your family's eating habits. You will also learn how to set the stage for change in your home and prepare your children for this "grow food" way of eating.

The dynamic duo for change is *love* and *fear:* Love for your children and fear of the Ds should be enough to get you started.

1. BECOME OBSESSED!

Here are some of the comments from parents who have used our NDD-Prevention Program successfully:

- "I realized I first had to become obsessed with feeding our family real food. That was the motivation I needed to get me going."

- "When I saw a child drinking a can of Coke, it actually hurt me inside, almost like when you see someone smoking a cigarette and wonder, 'Why is that person hurting himself?'"

- "Once I understood what fake food did to my child, I went through a stage of being an overprotective mother, as if fake food would put my child in danger. When she reached for it in the supermarket, my protective instinct went into overdrive. Before I knew about NDD, it didn't bother me. I didn't know any better. It helped me to go through that initial stage of being overprotective, and then I gradually learned to settle down a bit."

- "Dr. Bill's concept of grow foods as good medicine for my child helped me imagine all the colorful foods as 'grow medicines,' and I felt I had to give them to my child, like I would any medicine the doctor prescribed."

How do you know if you're there yet?

- You enter a supermarket and instinctively go directly to the grow-foods section on the perimeter.

- You "hurt" inside when you see a child wolfing down a Twinkie.

- Your child starts to grab a junk-food item at a buffet line and your protective instinct clicks in as if you sense danger.

- You feel joy seeing your children eat real foods.

From one mother: "*Be intentional. We tend to get so busy in life that we don't make healthy eating a priority.*"

2. AVOID THE BAD WORDS ON NUTRITION LABELS

The easiest way to separate junk food from real food is to avoid foods containing the following artificial additives:

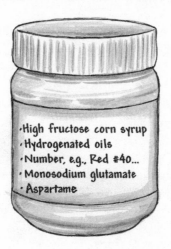

- High fructose corn syrup
- Hydrogenated oils
- Number, e.g., Red #40...
- Monosodium glutamate
- Aspartame

If you avoid foods containing these foolish five, you're already about 90 percent pure. Not only are these additives harmful to your family's health, they are guilty by association. As a general rule, if a packaged food contains any of these chemicals, the rest of the ingredients are nutritionally suspect.

Kids like label games. Play I Spy with My Little Eye and look for the bad word on the label. Keep junk foods with these bad words out of your house. Out of sight is out of mind and out of tummy.

From one mother: *"As the mother of three boys, I feel like I fight a daily war against junk food. I have found my daily battles are much easier if I keep junk food out of my home. It's much more difficult to have a temper tantrum over something that is not there to begin with."*

When bad words on food labels bother you, you are ready to prepare your family.

REAL FOOD VS. FAKE FOOD – A REMINDER

Here's an overview of the qualities of real foods, which prevent the Ds, and of the fake foods, which cause the Ds.

Real Foods

Fill without being fattening. Real foods have a built-in perk called a *high satiety factor,* which means they fill you up with fewer calories. Portion control is built in. You don't have to be the food police. Within reason, you can let your children eat as much as they want and as often as they want.

Satisfy hunger more. Because of the built-in satiety factor, real foods keep the child satisfied longer.

Balance blood sugar. Remember, as you learned on page 42, the brain behaves best when the blood sugar is steady.

Keep you healthy. The phytonutrients in real foods boost the immune system and help your growing child muster up his own internal medicine.

Fake Foods

Fatten without being filling. Fake foods have a *low satiety factor,* which means you need to overeat to feel satisfied. Fake foods require you to preach portion control, which takes the fun out of eating and invites rebellion.

Satisfy hunger less. Children get hungrier sooner, especially when eating high-carb foods.

Put blood sugar out of balance. Remember, the brain behaves worse when the blood sugar is erratic.

Make you sick. Fake foods weaken the immune system.

(Continued)

REAL FOOD VS. FAKE FOOD – A REMINDER *(CONT'D)*

Real Foods	Fake Foods
Make you smart. The grow foods on page 78 help the brain grow and function optimally. Real foods are *smart* foods.	**Make you less smart.** Fake foods can keep the developing brain from reaching its fullest potential. Fake foods are *dumb* foods.
Cost less. Healthier children get fewer Ds and you spend less on doctors.	**Cost more.** Sicker children means you spend more on doctors.
Help you live longer and healthier. Your grandchildren will thank you.	**Cause more diseases and an earlier death.** Your grandchildren will miss you.

---

3. PRACTICE THE "WE PRINCIPLE"

The "we principle" ("This is what *we* eat . . .") should flow as a natural part of parenting: "This is what we believe . . . , this is how we dress . . . , this is how we talk . . . , and this is what we eat." Children expect this guidance from their parents. Some motivated moms conclude that they shouldn't have to apologize to their children for making these changes: "After all, we're the parents, and we simply say, 'This is what we eat in our family — period.'"

"But, Mommy," Suzy protests, "my friends get to drink a lot of soda at their houses." "Sorry, honey, we don't drink that in our home," you might reply. And you might add a softer touch, "Because I love you, I can't let you pollute your beautiful brain and body with that junk."

And it's important not to be a nutritional wimp. One Mother's Day at our church, kids were asked to stand up and give a testimony to the influence their mothers had on their lives. Our son Dr. Bob volunteered, "I remember Mom serving us healthy food and not giving us a choice. We didn't question it, because there were no other options. We just learned to eat everything that was served. Thanks, Mom, for helping me learn to enjoy so many different foods."

It's all about attitude. As much as possible, try to keep a relaxed attitude about the change in family eating habits. The same goes for food shopping. If you buy it, they will eat it.

From one mother: *"Parents often feed their children with the expectation that they won't like vegetables or other healthy foods. Children have a remarkable ability to meet expectations. A negative attitude will never give broccoli a fair chance."*

And don't be a short-order cook. Make it clear to your kids that you expect them to eat the meals that you prepare.

From one mother: *"Baby food is simply mushed adult food served in smaller portions. Kids' meals should simply be adult real-food meals served in kid portions and with kid creations. Same food, same seasonings, and so on."*

---

4. PLAY SHOW-AND-TELL

Have the talk. If your children are preschool age and you're going to NDD-proof your home, you don't have to explain it; just do it. But if your children are older, set in their D-producing dietary ways, they might protest a kitchen makeover, so you might need to talk to them. Just as you don't leave sex education to the norms of the neighborhood, neither should you defer the responsibility for nutritional education. If your child is doing a presentation or science project at school, suggest one like "Smart Foods: Which Foods Are Best for Your Brain?"

Play Show-and-Tell. Explain the nutrients in grow foods to your kids so they'll value this term. Here's a sample dialogue: "Grow foods are filled with *protein,* which is like the steel, bricks, and concrete that construction workers use to build a strong building. Grow foods have *good carbs,* or good sugars, which provide energy for you to run, think, and learn. These foods have *smart fats,* which make your brain smart and your skin smooth. And grow foods are filled with *fiber,* which cleans out your body and makes your poop softer. Grow foods are packed with tiny foods called *vitamins* and *minerals* that act like energy batteries to help all the rest of the nutrients work better and help you grow. And they taste good!" Show your children the illustration on page 92 of a child's a clogged artery and tell them this child doesn't get enough blood flow to his brain, so he can't think as well at school. Tell them how his muscles don't get enough blood and energy, so he can't run fast for soccer, jump high for volleyball, or dance for very long.

Model healthy eating habits for your children. Tell them that you realize you need to have more energy to do better at work, so the whole family is going to start eating real food.

After you tell, show. Leave colorful grow-food bowls of fruits and veggies strategically placed throughout your home. Food in sight becomes food in tummy. Your child gets the message: "This is what we eat." Children watch what you eat and will eventually eat the same, just like they watch how you talk and eventually speak the words you speak.

Make your home compete with television messages. Place "ads" for grow foods all over your house. Now that TIVO-ers are able to fast-forward through ads during a recorded program, advertisers are working their junk-food ads into programs so that viewers have to see them. You can see this product placement (the old term was *hidden persuaders*) while Simon drinks a Coke during *American Idol.* Product placement within programs is one of the fastest-growing areas of TV advertising.

Kids conclude that it's cool to drink Coke because Simon says, or at least Simon shows. This form of advertising is actually more damaging to children than straight advertising because it gives children the message: "This is what celebrities eat and drink" — an unhealthy "we principle" you don't want to have in your home.

In the home environment, parents have to be more persuasive than television producers. It works on TV, so why not try it in the home? Surround your child with healthful messages: Display bowls of fruits and veggies and other healthy nibbles all through the house for snacking. Drink water, make a fruit-and-yogurt smoothie in the morning, enjoy whole wheat bread, and so on, and your child will get the healthy message.

SHOCK STATEMENTS

I "advertise" to kids in my pediatric office. Because there are some parents who still don't get it, I have to resort to shock statements. Next to the checkout counter, I display several large soda bottles that make the point:

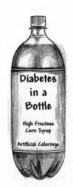

Enjoy a family kitchen makeover. Here is an opportunity to play Show-and-Tell and teach your children how to tell real foods from junk foods. Get a big box and go into the pantry with your kids. Start cleaning out the junk food. Then de-junk the fridge. In my office I tell children: "Go into your pantry and kitchen and pick out all the foods with any of the three bad words on the label. (See the five bad words on page 69.) Put these foods in a box and tell Mommy and Daddy that Dr. Bill says you get twenty-five cents for each bad word you spot."

From one mother: *"As we were doing our kitchen makeover, I explained that once the junk food was gone, I was no longer going to buy it. I explained that Mommy was learning about how grow foods, like fruits and vegetables, make us strong and healthy, and how sugary foods have been making us sick. Just like we wouldn't allow bad people into our homes to hurt us, we were no longer going to allow bad food into our home and bodies to hurt us."*

Take advantage of teachable moments. "Why did Grandpa have a heart attack?" your child might wonder. "Grandpa made poor food choices," you respectfully answer. When I got colon cancer from my earlier years of junk-food indulgences, and my kids asked why, Martha would respond, "Daddy made poor food choices." Fast-forward this scene ten years after cancer. One day a friend said to one of my children, "Your dad looks so healthy!" Our daughter Hayden responded, "Now he makes healthier food choices."

We often underestimate how much children understand of nutritional lessons. One day I was explaining to nine-year-old Jacob how fake fats clog arteries. Wanting to know how much of my preaching got through to him, I asked Jacob to write me a letter. Here's what Jacob wrote:

"Hydrogenated fats are bad fats. They inject foods with hydrogen so they can sit on the shelves. Then in a few years you can say, 'Look it's the doughnuts we got three years ago! They look as good as new.' Hydrogenated fats clog up your arteries. My grandpa had this sort of problem. He died when he was fifty-five years old, before I was born. It's good to have foods last a long time, but how long your body lasts is a lot more important than how long your food lasts. I wish I had my grandpa."

5. GIVE REAL FOODS KID-FRIENDLY NAMES

Kids do not like food restrictions, and the older they are, the less cooperative they're likely to be. Use the term *real food* or *grow food,* not *healthy food.* Older kids may equate healthy with icky. Rather than pontificate, "We're going to start eating healthy in our family" or "We're not going to have junk food in the house anymore," you'll get a lot more acceptance and cooperation if you present the change in a more positive way. Simply meet children where they are. Kid foods need kid names. Get behind the eyes of your child and imagine how they perceive "grow foods." Most likely they see these foods as *performance foods,* helping them to grow taller, smarter, prettier, and happier and to run faster. Or, you could relate these foods to what your child is into at a certain stage. "You're starting soccer next month, so we're going to start eating more soccer foods." Call these foods "baseball foods," "football foods," "dance foods," or "pretty hair foods." Real foods need real messages to get them into the minds and the mouths of children. Remember, makeovers work when presented in a positive way so that children feel that the makeover is better for them.

During a recent sports physical, I asked thirteen-year-old Jason if he had any concerns about his body. He volunteered, "Why am I so short?" Jason was a "late bloomer" who hadn't yet enjoyed the usual teen growth spurt. His nutrition was atrocious. Ah, a teachable moment! After explaining the relationship between grow foods and growth, I called them "tall foods." He got it! As he was leaving my office, Jason said, "I'm going to eat more tall foods."

From one mother: *"We call strawberries and blueberries 'nature's candy.' Fruit like apples and bananas are 'appetizers.' We make the names of good foods more exciting than those of fake foods. Healthy juice (such as Naked Juice) can be 'superman juice,' since it makes you feel so super."*

---

6. TEACH TRAFFIC-LIGHT EATING

Traffic-light eating is one of the most time-honored ways of getting grow foods into your kids. We use this simple way of teaching food choices in our family and our pediatric practice. Families find it fun.

Go Green-Light Foods

The green-light foods are go-for-it grow foods. Foods make our green-light list because:

- They are real.

- They are *filling,* so children are unlikely to overeat them.

- They are *nutrient-dense,* meaning they pack a lot of nutrition per calorie.

- The carbs in them are "good carbs," partnered with one or two friends (fiber and protein).

TRAFFIC-LIGHT LIST

Green-Light Foods	Yellow-Light Foods	Red-Light Foods
Good-for-you grow foods; "eat anytime" and enjoy.	*Slow down; enjoy, but not too often; "sometimes" foods.*	*Stop and think about a healthier choice. "We don't eat these in our family."*
All fruits	Butter	Beverages pre-sweetened with sugar or corn syrup
All veggies	Cookies, homemade	Cottonseed oil
Eggs	Frozen yogurt	Dyes
Flaxseed oil	Fruit juice, 100%	Foods with artificial sweeteners
Meat, lean	Honey	Foods with hydrogenated oils
Milk and cheese, low-fat	Meats, fatty	Prepackaged bakery goods
Nuts and seeds	Pasta	Gelatin desserts
Nut butters	Pastries, homemade	Marshmallows
Olive oil	White bread	Foods containing nitrates, e.g., some meats
Salmon		
Soy foods, e.g., tofu		
Whole grains		
Yogurt, organic		

- They are versatile. You can serve them many ways.

- They are free of harmful chemical additives.

- Kids like them! Real foods really are more flavorful.

Make green-light foods 90 percent of your shopping list. To get your children to go for more green-light foods, try these tips:

Market green-light foods. Display these foods prominently around your house. Head right for the green-light sections of the supermarket. (For tips on green-light shopping, see chapter 9.) When you eat out, go straight to the salad bar. That's where the green-light grow foods are.

Forget the math. One good thing about green-light foods is that *you don't have to count calories.* Children seldom overeat real food. Here's a simple guide to how many servings of green-light foods (such as the sixteen superfoods listed on page 99) your child should be eating:

Nine a day is nice.
Twelve a day is terrific.

How much is a serving? you might wonder. This depends upon your child's age. As a general rule, *one fistful of a food equals a serving.* Or, in the case of single foods, one egg, one apple, one tomato, and so on. Remember, children have much smaller fists than adults.

Play dress-up. It may require time, patience, and creative marketing to get more green-light foods past taste buds that have grown up with red- and yellow-light foods. Your family is more likely to accept this change if you go out of your way to make food taste better and serve it in a more attractive kid-friendly way. For creative feeding tips, see Make Meals More Fun, page 117.

Limit Yellow-Light Foods

Yellow-light foods make up the other 10 percent of the daily real-food diet. These foods are *treats* and *desserts,* "sometimes"

PREVENT "PASTA POT"

Most pastas should be yellow-light foods. Overdosing on pasta is a frequent contributor to children being overfat, especially around the middle. Serve *green-light* pasta: whole-grain pasta in smaller amounts and with a healthy sauce.

---

foods, and they are unhealthy only *in excess.* Some should *never be eaten alone,* but should be eaten with or following a green-light food. If you wonder why we put pasta in the yellow category, it's because in my experience pasta is the food children are most likely to overdose on, especially when it's smothered with fatty sauce. Plus, most pasta served is not whole grain. But a fistful of whole-grain pasta with cut-up veggies and a couple tablespoons of tomato sauce upgrades it to a green-light food. Similarly, a pie made at home with a whole-grain crust and whole fruit and sweetened with raisins, dates, or fruit concentrate gets close to being a green-light food.

It's okay to be a 90/10 family. While raising a "pure child" ideally means feeding her 100 percent green-light foods, this is seldom realistic or even desirable in many families. In fact, 90 percent green-light foods and 10 percent yellow-light foods is a diet that's more likely to be accepted by your child, who won't rebel from too many food restrictions. The good news is, if you shape young tastes early on, your child usually won't overdose on yellow-light foods and may not even be able to stomach red-light foods. Kids will always find their way to junk food, but if you can fill their growing bodies with as many grow foods as possible, there won't be much room left for junk.

Stop Red-Light Foods

Red-light foods are foods that say, "Stop and think! Could you make a healthier choice?" Red-light foods follow the "we principle": "We don't eat these in our family." Red-light foods are bad-for-you foods. They contribute to the Ds. They are:

- less filling, so children overeat them
- nutrient poor, with few nutrients per calorie
- fast carbs, which rush into the bloodstream because they have no friends to slow them down

In my practice I insist that my patients just not give their children red-light foods. We simply have to do something about the Ds. As a perk, children who are taught traffic-light eating often wind up monitoring their parents' eating habits. For example, a mother proudly told me, "The other night our seven-year-old said, 'Daddy, you shouldn't eat that. It's a red-light food.'"

From one mother: *"I feel my kids deserve an explanation rather than just a no. When we walk by candy machines or in a place with red-light foods and they ask for them, I always acknowledge their feelings by saying, 'You are right, they taste good. But they're not good for our bodies.' They're nearly always satisfied with that response and ready to move on."*

Most schools get a D in traffic-light eating, and as a result, students get the Ds. Once mothers become convinced of the harmful effects of red-light foods, their natural protective instinct goes on "red alert" and they appropriately protect their children from D-causing foods at school. Get involved in your school's PTA and push for healthier school cafeteria fare. I'm encouraged by a recent survey by *Reader's Digest* showing that 50 percent of mothers pack their children's school lunches.

CLUES THAT A FOOD CONTRIBUTES TO NDD

- You can't pronounce some of the added ingredients.
- The five bad words appear in the ingredients list: high fructose corn syrup, hydrogenated, monosodium glutamate, aspartame, and a # symbol.
- Eye-grabbing clichés such as "fit" and "lite" appear on the package. These terms often mean "lite" on nutrition and "unfit" for human consumption. With some foods, such as yogurt, the longer the ingredients list, the faker the food.
- The food is sold in the *center aisles* of the supermarket rather than around the perimeter.
- There are cartoon or movie characters hyping the product. What does Darth Vader know about your child's nutritional needs?

7. PRACTICE THE PILLS/SKILLS MIND-SET

More children are taking more pills for more illnesses than ever before. There are pills to perk them up, pills to calm them down, pills to help them focus, pills to help them sleep. If kids were first treated for NDD, they wouldn't need so many pills.

The longer I practice medicine, the more I realize that the most effective and scientific way to practice pediatrics is to teach parents and children the tools they need to manage their bodies. You will learn ways throughout this book to help your children muster up their own internal medicine. In practicing what I call the "pills/skills mind-set," instead of, or in addition to, asking the doctor, "What can my child *take?*" you ask, "What can my child *do?*" As soon as you change the "take" to "do," you prompt your child's doctor to click into a healthier mind-set, not "Here's what I *prescribe*" but "Here's what I *advise.*" The pills/skills approach is especially effective for preventing the Ds.

THE HOLE

Pills can cause a problem that I dub "the hole." Here's how kids get into the hole. A child is prescribed a perk-up pill, such as an antidepressant. "I think he's better," parents report. So the doctor leaves the child on the pill. After a few months on the pill, the brain habituates to, or gets used to, the pill, and the effect wears off. Or the brain gets used to the pill producing an antidepressant effect, so the brain decreases its own production of happy hormones, a drug effect called *down regulation.* The wise doctor tries to take the patient off the pill. The child gets worse. Here's the hole. Does the child get worse off the pill because he needs the pill, or is the getting worse really a withdrawal effect from the pill? There is often no way to tell.

The doctor is in the hole, and so are the parents and child. So the child goes back on the pill — and stays on it for years — or the dose is increased, or more pills are added to counteract the unpleasant side effects of the first pill. The only way for everyone to get out of the hole is to do what is called a *washout,* which means taking the child off all pills for at least six weeks to see which symptoms are caused by the problem and which are caused by the pills. During a washout, the child may experience unpleasant withdrawal effects, such as anxiety, depression, sleeplessness, and mood swings. It hurts to get out of the hole, but a washout is often the only way to tell whether or not a child still needs the medicines. It's best not to get into the hole in the first place.

In more than forty years in the practice of medicine, I have never seen a D that responded to the pills-only treatment. A safe and lasting treatment for any illness is either the skills-only approach or the pills/skills approach, but never pills only.

How I Use the Pills/Skills Model

I use the pills/skills model of medical care in approaching all the Ds in children. Here's an example of how I use it to help a child with ADHD (attention deficit/hyperactivity disorder). Jimmy and his parents are sitting in my office, and, based on the history of Jimmy's school performance provided by his teachers and parents and through my own assessment, I make the diagnosis of ADHD. I draw a graph for Jimmy's parents, like the one below.

I impress upon them that this is the healthiest way to approach any medical problem. First I teach them that ADHD is not really a disorder, it's a difference. Jimmy thinks, acts, and learns differently, so he needs a different style of teaching and parenting. He's simply quirky. I reassure them that the brains of many quirky kids are wired differently. They think outside the box. I tell them that with early intervention using the pills/skills model, they can channel their child's individual way of thinking to his advantage so

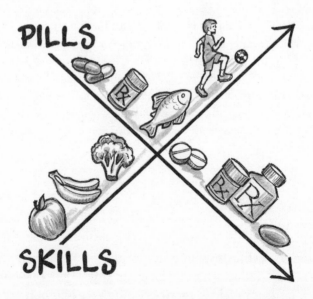

that he will continue to think outside the box and someday build a better box. The world is a better place because of quirky brains doing interesting things — think Mozart, Edison, Einstein, Bill Gates. Can you imagine what would have happened to Mozart's magical melodies had he been drugged? Yet if he had had early intervention and help, he might have lived much longer. Now that his parents understand Jimmy's quirk in a more positive way, here's what I advise:

Step 1: Practice the skills. I explain that NDD could be playing into Jimmy's ADHD. I give my NDD prescription from part 2 of this book (see page 97). I instruct them to keep a diary and document the changes they've made. In addition to practicing new nutritional skills, I recommend educational skills such as tutoring, behavior modification, matching child and teacher, etc. Then I reevaluate the situation in about three weeks to determine if any progress has been made.

Step 2: Possibly add pills. Suppose Jimmy is making progress, but Jimmy's parents, his teacher, and perhaps an ADHD specialist feel he is still struggling and might benefit from pills. I prescribe the pills using the "start low, go slow" approach, starting with a low dose and gradually increasing if necessary. I impress upon the parents that the pills are to be used *in addition to,* not instead of the skills. And, to reinforce the fact that the skills are more important than the pills, I tell them, "When you come back in a month for a 'medication check,' bring your diary. I will only refill the prescription of the pills if you assure me that you have practiced the skills."

I make this pills/skills deal with the parents because I don't want Jimmy to begin life with the "have a problem, pop a pill" mind-set. Rather, I want children to learn early on how to take control of their quirks and practice the pills/skills mind-set throughout their lives.

8. PREVENT ANOTHER NDD: NATURE DEFICIT DISORDER

Once upon a time children ran around outside for exercise and entertainment. Nowadays they sit indoors in front of a screen for entertainment, and perhaps exercise their tiny eye and finger

---

MDD – MOVEMENT DEFICIT DISORDER

MDD can lead to NDD. We have an NDD-prevention policy in our home: Sitting equals moving. Kids need to spend at least as much time moving as they do sitting. When children began sitting rather than running for entertainment, the number of Ds increased. Any correlation? Science says yes:

- In a revealing study, boys labeled with ADD were divided into two groups. One group got an extra twenty minutes a day of "prescribed" vigorous exercise; the other group didn't. Compared with the "sitters," the "movers" showed remarkable improvement in their ADD, especially in their ability to sit still and focus, and they required fewer drugs.
- Increased movement of the body increases blood flow to the brain. Neuroscientists have found that movement is great "grow food" for the brain. Increased blood flow to the brain increases the release of a substance called nerve growth factor, or NGF, which is like Miracle-Gro for the brain.
- Movement mellows the mind. Increased blood flow to the brain releases "happy hormones," nature's own antidepressants and anti-anxiety medicines.

Recess vs. Ritalin

Heather, a nine-year-old in our pediatric practice, was misdiagnosed with ADD and a learning disability because she had diffi-

muscles — and get sicker, sadder, and fatter. Modern kids have a green-grass deficiency. What drug do they need? The great outdoors. The sights and sounds of nature both relax the mind and invigorate the body. The colors, the movement, the fresh air, and the sun's energy are just what the D doctor ordered.

Our family hobby is sailing. When I realized that our children

culty spelling. Here is the treatment I prescribed: "Have her jump on a home mini-trampoline while someone coaches her on her spelling homework." After this rather unconventional movement therapy, her spelling improved.

Motivate your school to move your child. When school administrators started taking away recess, school nurses started giving more Ritalin. Any correlation? Join the PTA and get your school focused on a movement toward recess. Twenty minutes of unstructured play is another remedy the D doctor ordered. Perhaps taking a brisk walk while enjoying some unstructured goofy behavior might settle the brain.

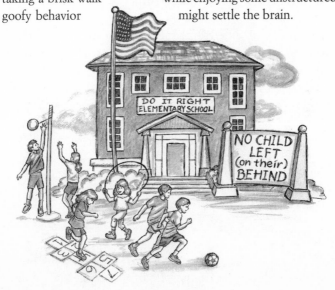

were suffering from Nature Deficit Disorder, our family therapy was to pile all the kids onto a rented sailboat in the Caribbean and sail around the islands. (Actually, it's a relatively economical family vacation.) We sailed it ourselves, just the family. Here's the catch. The kids were not allowed to bring along any electronics: no computers, no iPods. After a day or so of withdrawal from being unplugged, they plugged into the attractions of nature, and it was *d*elightful. Studies show exposure to sunlight and fresh air improves attention and learning.

The bottom line: If your child is labeled with ADD, OCD, or any other D that demands drugs, take her for a walk in the park rather than for a ride to the drugstore.

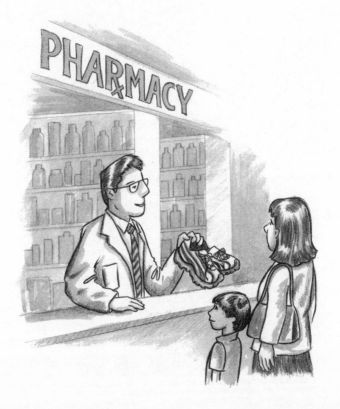

9. NO EXCUSES, PLEASE!

Here are the top excuses I hear from parents who continue to feed their children junk food:

"It's less expensive." Actually, it's *more expensive* to feed your children fake food than wholesome food. When it comes to real food, you get what you pay for: wellness. While it is true that wholesome food sometimes costs more than junk food at the checkout counter, consider the money-saving effects of healthful food: You're likely to miss less work, because your child is likely to be sick less often. You are likely to have fewer doctor bills, because wholesome food builds your child's immune system. Those two reasons alone will probably save you much more money than the extra you spend on nutritious foods. Also, think of feeding your child nutritious foods as an investment in your child's future, one of the most valuable bequests you can give — the gift of health.

Here are some suggestions for how to get more for less if you're on a tight food-shopping budget:

- Buy in bulk and split the cost with another family.

- Buy in bulk from food co-ops.

- Watch Sunday newspapers for coupons and sales.

- Grow your own fruits and vegetables.

- Buy more when on sale and in season and freeze.

- During berry-picking season, pick pounds of them and store them in your freezer.

- Patronize your local farmer's market and "real food" stores. The higher their sales volume, the lower their prices will be.

- Think quality, not quantity. Kids eat much more of nonfilling "fluff" foods than they do of nutrient-dense grow foods.

Pay the supermarket *farm*acy now or the D doctor later.

"But my children won't eat healthy foods." Yes, they will. It's a matter of presentation and marketing. If you buy and serve only wholesome foods, they will eat them. This has been proven in food-refusal studies at the nutrition laboratory at Penn State University, where children who refused to eat certain foods were studied. Researchers found that the children did eventually eat the refused food, such as broccoli and greens, but it took fifteen to twenty times of presenting these foods before they became familiar enough for the children to be willing to eat them. If there is no other choice, and if they are hungry enough, children will eat the foods you give them.

From one mother: "After I read that a toddler might need to be exposed to a food fifteen or more times until he or she tries it, and that most parents give up after four or five tries, we added a small 'no, thank you' plate to our toddler's place setting. We continued to offer him the 'unpopular' vegetables but told him that if he didn't want to eat them, he could set it on the 'no, thank you' plate. We noticed that he'll eventually try the foods — sometimes even changing his mind and taking it off the 'no, thank you' plate in the middle of a meal."

"But it takes time to prepare healthful foods." While you might think it takes you less time to serve fast, fake foods, it actually wastes time in the long run. When you consider the time spent taking your child to doctors and handling missed work, you'll see that wellness is less time-consuming than illness.

"But junk food doesn't seem to bother my child." On the outside, some children appear impervious to the D-producing effects of fake food, but they can be sick on the inside. Illness has a way of sneaking up on a young person. New research is showing that dementia, even Alzheimer's, actually begins in childhood.

Your children need you to help them make wise food choices. Children don't think in the future. They do not think, "I ate a bunch of hot dogs now, so my heart is going to stop beating sooner." They think in the present. You need to be the adult in this situation and think like an adult. Your child needs you to do this. *No excuses, just do it!* Your children will later thank you for it.

10. TAKE YOUR CHILD ON A FOOD PATH THROUGH THE BODY

In the previous chapter, you learned how NDD affects the brain. Yet, nutritional deficit disorder affects every part of a child's growing body. Following a food path through your child's body is a fun way to teach her about grow foods. Here's a way to explain what is happening in her body.

Grow a Healthy Heart

"Your heart pumps blood into the rivers of blood vessels that flow all through your body. The blood delivers energy for you to play and food for you to grow. Think of your blood vessels as rivers and creeks. When you dump garbage in rivers, the water gets muddy and dirty. When you eat junk food, you dump garbage into your blood vessels. Look at the picture below of a blood vessel from a person who ate too much junk food. When the junk food gets into your blood, it acts like sticky stuff or like the garbage in a muddy river. Over many years this sticky stuff piles up, like junk piles up on river banks, and makes the blood flow more slowly, so you don't get enough energy in your body to think smart, run fast, or play soccer well.

"Now look at the arteries of a child who ate grow foods, like fruits, veggies, fish, greens, and beans. This child has blood like clean rivers and arteries like a Slip 'N Slide.

"Which arteries do you want to have?"

Once your child understands the concept of how grow foods create smooth arteries, and junk foods dump sticky stuff, like pollution, into these "rivers," go to the next lesson.

"Once upon a time, even doctors thought our blood vessels were just like a rubber hose: Blood comes in one end and goes out the other, and nothing else happens. Now we know that the lining of our blood vessels [point to the picture] has millions of magical glands, like tiny squirt bottles. These glands make *magical juices* from your body's own chemistry set that squirt smart medicines into the rivers of your bloodstream to make you smart and strong.

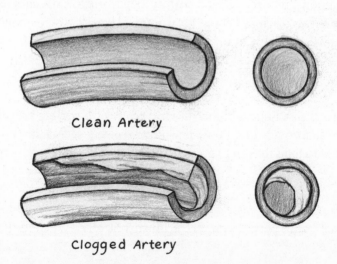

Clean Artery

Clogged Artery

But if you eat lots of junk food, that sticky stuff piles up and damages these tiny squirt bottles, so they can't work. When Dr. Bill tells you he wants you to muster up your own internal medicine, such as for your ADD, this is what he means. This is where your internal medicine comes from. That's why we have to feed the lining of our arteries right.

"Guess how to get these glands, or squirt bottles, to open and squirt the magical medicines into your bloodstream. By moving! When you run, dance, or play outside, your blood flows faster across these glands and opens the lids on these bottles, letting more medicine out, sort of like a highway surface with a self-maintenance crew. That's how movement musters up your own internal medicine."

Note to Mom and Dad: The endothelium, or lining of the blood vessels, is the body's largest endocrine system. The magical medicines provided by the endothelium are the "anti" disease substances you need, such as antidepressants, antihypertensives, anti-Alzheimer's, and so on. These natural internal medicines also lower the "highs," such as high blood pressure, high blood sugar, and high cholesterol. Help your children appreciate that the lining of the blood vessels is like their own personal doctor inside, and the more they listen to their doctor, the healthier they will grow. Preventing NDD and MDD (movement deficit disorder, see page 86) helps grow a healthy endothelium.

If your child is in high school and studying biology, you could create a very informative science project for the whole family. Do an online search for *endothelial function* (medical jargon for what the lining of the blood vessels does).

Grow a Smarter Brain

"Your brain uses more of the food you eat than any other part of your body does. If you put smart food into your brain, like

What's in your arteries?

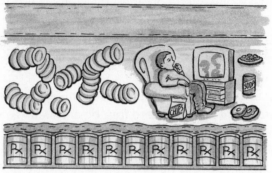

Sticky stuff, rough edges, endothelial d<u>y</u>sfunction

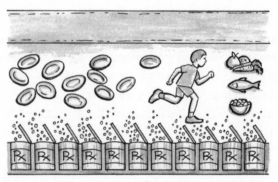

Easy blood flow, smooth edges, healthy endothelium

salmon, blueberries, and spinach, you can pay better attention and get better grades at school. But because your brain uses so much of the food you eat, it can run out of fuel fast. That's why it's smart to start the day with a brainy breakfast and nibble on the smart foods that I pack for your snacks. Here's how the smart foods help your brain grow to be smart.

"Think of your brain as a giant computer with lots of electrical wires inside. How fast your computer runs, or how well you can think and learn, depends on how fast those electrical wires fire. See that lamp cord over there? Feel the wire. That rubbery stuff is called insulation. It helps the electricity inside flow better. If that wire didn't have good insulation on it, it wouldn't work as well and the light wouldn't shine so brightly. The same thing happens in your brain. When you eat smart foods, the insulation around the electrical wires in your brain works better so your brain can shine brighter just like the lightbulb. Grow foods grow good insulation in your brain so you can think smarter.

"What foods do you want to feed your brain?"

Leave Your Children a Lifelong Legacy

What's in your will? Money and stuff you want your children to inherit? Consider a more valuable inheritance, one that every parent, no matter what their economic situation, can leave their children and grandchildren: *health.*

One day a mother in my office asked me how she could change her husband's eating habits because he often sabotaged the changes she was trying to make in their family's eating. I asked, "What's his profession?" "He's an investment banker," she replied. "Good, tonight I'm giving a talk on healthful eating to a parent group at a local school. Tell him Dr. Bill is giving a talk entitled "The Best Long-Term Investment You Can Make for Your Family."

Early in my talk I could see him squirming, as if thinking, "He's talking about *food,* not money." As I got deeper into how early eating habits affect later health and how kids are likely to pass on to their own kids the eating habits they grew up with, I noticed Mr. Investment Banker was riveted to my message. After the talk, he thanked me for opening his eyes to this family "investment."

Now that you know the ten simple steps to getting started, let's move on to Dr. Bill's prescription for preventing NDD.

II

Dr. Sears's Prescription: Seven Simple Steps to Prevent NDD

In part 1 you learned why you must make some changes in your family's diet. In part 2 you will learn how. *Now that you are informed, motivated, afraid, obsessed, or whatever it takes to make you a real-food believer, here are the seven simple steps to preventing NDD:*

1. *Feed your family grow foods.*
2. *Reshape young tastes.*
3. *Begin the day with a brainy breakfast.*
4. *Raise a grazer.*
5. *Encourage healthy eating while out and at school.*
6. *Raise a supermarket-savvy shopper.*
7. *Supplement, if necessary.*

The magic word in child development is thrive. *All kids grow, which simply means they get bigger and heavier. Kids even grow on junk food. But they don't thrive on junk food, which means they don't grow to be the best they can be physically, intellectually, and emotionally. We want our children to thrive, and that's what these seven simple steps are designed to do.*

4

Step 1: Feed Your Family Grow Foods

Now that you are ready to make over your family's eating habits, let's begin with getting your kids used to eating real foods, especially those sixteen superfoods that are the most NDD-preventing. Call them "grow foods."

THE SUPER SIXTEEN VS. THE SICK SIXTEEN

Parents, be honest. Check off how many of the sixteen superfoods and how many of the sixteen sick foods your family eats regularly. Which checklist is longer? If the real-foods list is longer, you are on the right track for preventing the Ds. If the sick-foods list is longer, your family is sick, and you need to make a change. The super sixteen are green-light foods. At least 90 percent of your family's diet should be from among these foods. The sick sixteen are red-light foods. None of these fake foods or chemicals belong in your kitchen.

The Super Sixteen

Avocados

Beef and turkey, lean, organic

"Blues": blueberries

Eggs

"Greens": spinach, arugula, chard, broccoli, bok choy

Nuts and nut butter

Oils: fish, flaxseed, olive

"Orange/yellows": carrots, papaya, mango, orange, apricots

"Pinks": grapefruit, guava

Potatoes, sweet potatoes, yams

"Reds": strawberries, watermelon, tomatoes, peppers, apples, kidney beans, lentils

Salmon, wild

Soy foods: edamame, soy nuts, tofu

Spices: cinnamon, turmeric

Whole grains: whole wheat, oats, wild rice, amaranth

Yogurt, organic

The Sick Sixteen

Artificial colorings: blue #1, blue #2, green #3, etc.

Artificial flavor enhancers: MSG, hydrolyzed vegetable protein (HVP)

Artificial preservatives: sulfites, nitrites, nitrates, BHA, BHT, sodium benzoate, benzoic acid

Artificial sweeteners: aspartame, sucralose, saccharin

Bakery bads (e.g., cupcakes, tarts, and Twinkies)

Beef jerky

Candy (except 70 percent dark chocolate treats)

Cereals with fewer than 3 grams protein, 3 grams fiber, and more than 6 grams added sugar per serving

Cottonseed oil

Gelatin desserts with artificial flavors and colors

High fructose corn syrup

Hydrogenated oils

Marshmallows

Shortcut foods: "lite," "fit," "quik"

Sweetened beverages

White bread

Healthy relatives of the super sixteen: bell peppers, chili peppers, purple grapes, melon, all berries, pomegranate juice, prunes, squash, kiwi, and sunflower seeds. Basically, *all fruits, vegetables, and whole grains belong on the grow-foods list.*

The super sixteen have in common:

- have spent none or minimal time in the food factory
- contain healthy fats
- are nutrient-dense: packed with more nutrition per calorie
- are brain- and immune-system boosting
- improve attention and learning
- shape young tastes in the right direction
- prevent the Ds

In a nutshell: These foods help keep your family healthy, happy, and lean.

On the other hand, the sick sixteen have the opposite in common:

- have spent more time in the food factory
- contain most unhealthy fats
- are less nutrient-dense
- weaken the immune system
- lessen attention and learning
- shape young tastes in the wrong direction
- cause the Ds

In a nutshell: These foods make your family sick, sad, and fat.

FEED YOUR FAMILY MORE FISH AND PHYTOS

Three important foods for preventing NDD are seafood, vegetables, and fruits. But fish and vegetables are the foods parents often find the most challenging to get their kids to eat. You will now learn creative ways to feed your child more of these top grow foods.

Vegetables are the ideal grow food. In fact, any food that itself has to grow helps your child grow. Plant a tomato seed and watch it become a healthy tomato. The seed absorbs nutrients from the soil and blossoms into a green plant. This flowering plant absorbs energy from the sun and feeds the nutrients to the tomato to help it grow. To protect itself from pests, the smart tomato makes medicines or phytonutrients (phytos) such as lycopene, which both fights disease and turns the tomato red. These phytos help your child grow strong and stay healthy. The more colorful the fruit or veggie, the more phyto-full the food. Many phyto-moms in our practice have shared with me, "Once I followed your advice of putting more color on my child's plate, he stopped getting sick as often."

Why Kids Need More Phytos

Oxidation is the biochemical exhaust from the metabolism of the body's engine. Yet, unlike our car engines, our bodies don't have exhaust pipes. So we need to eat anti-exhaust nutrients — antioxidants such as phytos — that internally mop up the exhaust. Otherwise this exhaust accumulates, especially in our immune system, and two things happen: We get sick more often and we "rust." In a nutshell, this is the process of aging.

Premature aging is how we doctors describe the epidemic of the body Ds among children. Here's why. Because growing children eat proportionally more food for their body weight than adults do (children use around 25 percent of the calories they eat just to grow), they produce proportionally more exhaust, or oxidation, from the food they eat. The brain uses at least 20 percent of all the oxygen a child breathes and around 25 percent of all the food energy a child consumes. As a result, the brain produces the most oxidation. Therefore, to prevent NDD, children need to eat more antioxidants, or phytos, than adults do. But they don't as a rule do so. Eating fewer phytos means more oxidation, which leads to more Ds. What's the solution? Kids need to eat more phytos.

Pure kids eat enough antioxidants to balance their oxidants. Junk-food kids, on the other hand, eat many more exhaust-producing foods and fewer anti-exhaust foods. As a result, their brains and bodies become *exhausted* or full of inflammation. That's how they become *iBods*. (For an explanation of the term *iBod*, see page 46).

Phyto Feeding Tips

Teach your children why phytos are good for them. Use language kids can relate to: "Phytos keep you from getting sick." "Phytos make your skin and hair pretty."

Make phytos fun. The grow foods listed on page 105 are full of phytos. While you want your children to grow up regarding real food as real medicine, appreciating that concept may be beyond the young child. Yet even a preschooler can learn that phytos fight germs. When asked what makes a tomato red, our five-year-old granddaughter, Ashton, proudly exclaims, "Lycopene!" When asked what makes a carrot orange, she exclaims, "Carotenoids!" When asked what makes a blueberry blue, she manages to mumble the tongue twister "anthocyanins." While she may be too young to really understand how phytos boost her immune system, at this impressionable age she is making the connection between *colorful foods* and *a beauty-full body.* When asked what carotenoids and lycopene do, she says, "They make me pretty and healthy." If you want to delve deeper into how phytos fight disease, see our website www.AskDrSears.com/phytos.

Phytos are stronger in combination. Grandmother was nutritionally correct when she advised, "Eat a variety of fruits and vegetables." When phytos partner with one another, they work better in the body through a biochemical principle called *synergy,* a sort of 1 + 1 = the disease-fighting effect of 3 or 4. Partner a blue with a red and the dynamic duo is more powerful than eating each one separately. In our kitchen we follow the "S-S-S Guide" — *smoothies, soups, and salads.* These dishes have a whole nutritional orchestra of phytos. Mother Nature is also a wise nutritionist. There are no fruits or vegetables that contain only one vitamin or one mineral. Every plant food has its own multivitamin/ multimineral combination. Again, the more color on a plate, the better the phytos fight the germs.

Eat phytos first. Back to Grandmother's nutritional wisdom: "Eat fruits and vegetables before dessert." Or, what we say nowadays in our family: "Eat grow foods before fun foods." The natural phytos, or antioxidants, in colorful foods like (pink) seafood, (blue) berries, and (red) apples blunt the effects of foods that throw the body out of biochemical balance. For example, when your teen eats a big salad before wolfing down a hamburger, the phytos in

---

Dr. Sears says: The principle of nutritional synergy explains why the three Ss — smoothies, soups, and salads — are healthy family meals.

the salad blunt some of the wear-and-tear effects of the processed beef and fake white bread. And piling lettuce, onions, and tomatoes on top of the burger makes it at least more biochemically acceptable to the body.

Once your family gets used to the idea that eating colorful foods is caring for the body, they are more likely to grab an apple or an orange as they rush past the grow-food bowl on the kitchen counter. If you plant in your child's mind the idea that the colors in plant foods are good for him, he will form a pattern of association. Then when he sees these colorful foods, it will trigger a reflex: "Gotta eat it!" This mindful eating may take time to instill in your children, but you will get there. I have seen this pattern occur hundreds of times in the "pure families" in my practice.

Eat phytos frequently. Phyto-containing fruits and veggies are nutritious snack foods. They are satisfying without being over-filling, and it's hard to overeat them. As an additional perk, many phytos are high in vitamin C. Because this vitamin is not stored in the body, it requires a steady intake.

How many phytos a day? Follow the "nine is nice" guide. One serving equals around one fist size, and nine handfuls of phytos a day should keep the D doctor away.

Juicy juices. Juices are a sweet way to get phytos into your kids. But most juices run a distant second to the real fruits and vegetables they are juiced from. Here are some top juices and tips for serving them:

- Pomegranate juice is full of phytos and a sweet favorite of children. Nutrition researchers who have studied various pomegranate juice brands say Pom Wonderful is the top nutritional favorite.

FIFTEEN FAVORITE PHYTO FOODS

Here are fifteen fruits and vegetables that are high in phytos (and that are liked by most children):

Apples	Legumes: beans, lentils
Asparagus	Oranges
Avocados	Papaya
Berries: blueberries, straw-	Pink grapefruit
berries	Red peppers
Broccoli	Spinach
Cherries	Sweet potatoes
Grapes: red, black	Tomatoes

- Green veggie juices. Our favorite is Essential Greens Veggie juice from Trader Joe's. It is higher in protein and fiber, vitamin C, calcium, and many phytos than other green juices.

- Prune juice is highest in iron, zinc, fiber, and niacin.

- Orange juice is highest in vitamin C; grapefruit juice is the second highest.

- White grape juice is the most intestines-friendly and a favorite when kids are on the "sips only" diet for diarrhea.

- Use pomegranate, carrot, and Essential Greens Veggie juices in your smoothies. (See our smoothie recipe, page 182.) Blend fruits and veggies into your smoothies rather than juicing them to retain more of the nutritious pulp.

- Dilute juice with half water. When serving juice as a substitute for water, use just enough of the child's favorite juice to color it.

- Avoid these cute words on juice container labels: "punch," "drink," and "cocktail." These unnutritious junk juices are usually full of artificial sweeteners and colors and are mostly water with very little juice. We rank them in the "bad for you" category. Instead, go for 100 percent juice.

- Avoid "see-through" juices, such as apple juice; the cloudy stuff, which contains most of the nutrients, has been removed.

- Avoid juices that contain preservatives such as sodium benzoate.

Go Fish!

These are the two most important words in preventing NDD. On page 25 you learned how omega-3 fats get into your child's brain to make it think better and into the tissues of his body to make it perform better. Omega 3s are to the brain what calcium is to the bones. I believe that *a deficiency of omega-3 fats is the number one nutritional problem in kids.* Fortunately, this deficiency is easily corrected.

In teaching families about fish, I call seafood the "head-to-toe nutrient." Studies show that families who eat more fish have a lower incidence of nearly all these Ds:

- ADD/ADHD
- allergic diseases: asthma, dermatitis, eczema
- BPD (bipolar disorder)

- cardiovascular disease
- depression
- diabetes
- eye diseases: improves visual acuity
- inflammatory bowel disease
- joint disease: arthritis
- learning disabilities

Simply put, children who eat more fish think better, see better, run better, feel better, and look better. I can't think of another nutrient that can do all of that. Seafood is the most nutrient-dense food you can feed your family. "Nutrient-dense" is the highest honor you could pay any food. Here's the nutritional profile of 3.5 ounces (an average serving for a school-age child) of a fillet of wild Alaskan salmon:

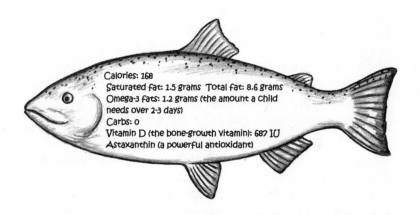

Calories: 168
Saturated fat: 1.5 grams Total fat: 8.6 grams
Omega-3 fats: 1.2 grams (the amount a child needs over 2-3 days)
Carbs: 0
Vitamin D (the bone-growth vitamin): 687 IU
Astaxanthin (a powerful antioxidant)

Questions You May Have About "Going Fishing"

How much fish should my child eat?

Shoot for three ounces of salmon at least two times a week for children under four and six ounces two times a week for adults and children over four years of age. Eating this amount of fish twice a week will give your children at least 50 percent of the omega-3 DHA they need.

Are the omega 3s in flaxseed oil just as good as the omega 3s in seafood?

Flaxseed oil (and flaxseed meal, which is ground flaxseeds) is a very healthy oil. I often "prescribe" a tablespoon of flaxseed oil added to a smoothie for children who actually need more nutrition from undereating. Even though flaxseed oil is labeled as an omega 3, it does not behave as well biochemically in the body as the omega 3s that come from seafood. In fact, none of the omega 3s found in plant sources (e.g., flaxseed oil, nuts and nut oils, and canola oil) are as rich as the omega 3s in seafood. Here's why.

The omega 3s found in flaxseed oil are called alphalinolenic acid. ALA is a shorter molecule, only eighteen carbons long, than the two omega 3s in seafood, eicosapentaenoic acid (EPA) and docosahexaenoic acid (DHA), which are twenty and twenty-two carbons long, respectively. When you eat plant sources of omega 3s, the body has to do a series of complex biochemical dances to add two or four carbons onto the "short guys" (the plant oils) to turn them into the longer EPA and DHA, or "tall guys," which are the omega 3s that the brain and the body actually use. How efficiently the body can do this carbon add-on conversion varies from person to person, especially in children. Studies estimate that only around 3 to 5 percent of the omega-3 oils found in plant oils are converted to the brain-building omega 3 DHA. The DHA and EPA omega 3s found in seafood are called preformed omega 3s, which means that the body doesn't have to change them to use them.

Buyer beware. Now that omega 3s are so popular, food packagers want to advertise them on their labels. Some food makers slip in some of the less expensive omega 3s, like flaxseed oil and canola oil, yet the package will say, "fortified with omega 3s." Look for a package label that says, "omega 3 DHA" or "omega 3s from marine sources."

How young can my children start eating salmon?

The best way to raise little fish eaters is to start early. In our family and in our pediatric practice we begin serving infants salmon at around nine months of age. Begin with a fingertipful of mushed salmon and increase the amount as your baby wishes. By shaping young tastes to like seafood, your child is likely to grow up to be a fish eater.

What if my child doesn't like fish?

It's all in the presentation. Serve it and they will eat it. Remember the "we principle" on page 71. Once children get the message that Mom serves salmon twice a week, they understand that "this is what we're supposed to eat." You can sneak salmon into your child's favorite foods: add it to casseroles, make salmon "meatballs" and spaghetti sauce, and serve salmon "fish sticks." If your child just won't eat seafood, then give her a daily omega-3 supplement (see page 167). And try the tasty seafood recipes on pages 188, 194, 195, and 197.

What about the mercury and other pollutants in seafood? I'm worried about the safety.

Because there has been a lot of scary information about seafood safety in the press, parents are naturally concerned. The general consensus among doctors and experts in seafood safety is, in a nutshell, "The health benefits of seafood far outweigh the risks."

It is safe to feed your family the following green-light "go fish" in the amounts recommended on page 108:

- wild Alaskan salmon
- non-albacore tuna
- sardines

Red-light "no fish" are:

- swordfish
- shark
- mackerel
- tile fish
- albacore tuna

A reliable source for safe and tasty fish is www.vitalchoice .com. Our family and patients in our practice have used this site for many years and have found it to be one of the best. Or visit the FDA's or the EPA's safe seafood website, www.cfsan.fda.gov/ seafood1.html or www.epa.gov/mercury.

Should I serve my child wild or farm-raised fish? Farm-raised fish is usually cheaper.

What's your child's health worth? Throughout this book you have learned that feeding your child pure food is actually less expensive in the long run. You've also learned that what the animal eats determines how healthy the food is. This is especially true with wild versus farm-raised fish. I have had the opportunity to look into the farmed-versus-wild question, and I have concluded that in our family and pediatric practice, wild fish, especially wild salmon, is better for several reasons.

Wild Alaskan salmon is higher in the good fats, lower in saturated fats, and higher in antioxidants or phytos. This makes sense because wild salmon eat healthy sea plants that themselves are high in the healthiest fat, omega 3s. Astaxanthin, the potent phyto or antioxidant that gives wild fish its pink color, occurs in very high levels in wild salmon. In some farmed seafood, the pink color is actually artificial food coloring.

Imagine this tale of two fish: The wild salmon swims thousands of miles (with strong muscles) and then eats what fish are programmed to eat (healthy sea plants). The wild fish can search all around for just the perfect food. The farmed fish sits around in a pen all day and eats junk food chosen by the fish farmer instead of the fish.

Consider this fish story, which was told to me by a fisherman. A favorite experiment among fisherman is to take a domestic or farm-raised fish and put it in the wild. The slow-to-grow farm-raised fish soon becomes a fast-growing wild fish. I have been told that this happens even when you take a goldfish out of the bowl and put him in an outside pond. How do you want your children to grow? Would you rather pay the fisherman now or the doctor later?

5

Step 2: Reshape Young Tastes

If your children have spent many years eating artificially sweetened, oversalted fake foods, their taste buds have been spoiled. Now that you have decided to be a "pure parent," it may take a while to reshape their tastes toward liking and then craving real food. Expect occasional resistance ("Oh, Mom's gone healthy again!"). It may take several weeks or months to gradually reshape your children's tastes to prefer real food, but it will happen. The cells lining the gut have the most rapid turnover rate in the whole body. Every few weeks your child's gut gets a new coating of cells. So, as she sloughs off the old cells — and the old food habits — hopefully, the new cells will welcome the upgraded cuisine. Researchers have found that three factors shape young tastes: what their parents and peers eat, the taste of the food, and the gut feelings (good or bad) the child has after eating. Try these taste-shaping tips:

START EARLY

The window of opportunity for shaping young tastes is open widest in the first few years. The earlier you start feeding your children a real-food diet, the easier it is to shape their tastes. Studies show that food choices made by toddlers are likely to persist. Around six months, go straight to feeding them real foods. Make your own baby food and toddler food. In fact, to nutrition-savvy moms, baby food and toddler food is simply the real food that the rest of the family eats but blended, pureed, and served in a consistency and portion appropriate to the child's age and stage of development.

Start small, go slow. For infants, start with a fingertipful and gradually increase to a teaspoon, then to a tablespoon.

Present it and they will eat it. With increasing age, children become increasingly reluctant to try new tastes and textures. Researchers even have a word for a reluctance to try new things, including new foods: *neophobia.* Long-term studies on children's food preferences have shown that the strongest predictor of the number of foods liked at eight years of age is the number of foods liked at four years of age. And newly tasted foods were more likely to be accepted between two and four years of age than between four and eight years of age. This study also showed that the strongest predictor of children's food preferences were the preferences of their mothers. If their mothers liked and ate certain foods, the children tended to copy. If their mothers tended to dislike and not eat certain foods, the children tended to copy those preferences and dislikes.

Try to introduce as many different foods with different tastes and textures as early on as possible. The best time for introducing lots of new foods is *between one and two years of age.* At this stage toddlers like to play copycat: you eat it, they want it too. This is when the intestinal lining of a two-year-old is mature enough to digest a wide variety of foods but the "gut brain" has not yet been shaped toward junk food. Parents, capitalize on this window of opportunity before the usual parent-child power struggles begin at two or three years of age.

From one mother: *"I believe that because I made all of her baby food myself, my daughter has become a more adventurous eater with a taste for real food. Jarred baby food tastes bland and awful! It is also imperative to set a good example, so I have a policy of not eating anything in front of my daughter that I wouldn't allow her to have. (She is going to ask for a bite of it!) It is definitely getting tougher, now that she is in preschool and she is aware that these other junk foods exist. By far the toughest part is not getting HER to eat healthy, but convincing OTHER PEOPLE not to give her junk. Her preschool still serves junk-flavored yogurt, so I'm currently lobbying them to switch to plain yogurt. Parents need to demand better food for their children and not give in!"*

DON'T FUSS OVER FOOD

You want your children to regard food as a fun and normal part of life, not something filled with restrictions and policing. It's all in the presentation. If you present real foods in a loving way and your child gets the message "My mom makes me eat broccoli because she really loves me and knows what's good for me," that's great, but if you sense that food is becoming an increasing battle, back off a bit. Above all, don't fuss over food portions or how much your child eats. Hungry children will eat. They come prewired for survival. And it's hard to overeat real food.

From accepting to liking to craving. Here's what you can expect when you follow this NDD-prevention prescription. First, your children will *accept* the family food makeover (possibly reluctantly, but they have no other choice). Then, after weeks — or months, depending on how long they have been eating fake foods — they will begin to *like* or even prefer real foods. Finally, they will reach the promised land of *craving* real foods because they experience a change in how they feel and perform.

From one mother: *"We tell our five-year-old that our tastes change as we get older, so just because he doesn't like something the first time doesn't mean he won't like it when he's older. Other adults have been pleasantly surprised by his positive attitude toward food when he says things like, 'Well I don't like that yet, but I will when I'm bigger.'"*

GO SLOWLY

While some families can go green overnight, many families, especially those with older children, need to reshape tastes gradually. Here are a couple of helpful tips:

- Instead of white bread, switch to 50 percent whole grain, then 80 percent, then 100 percent.

- Serve plain yogurt, but sweeten it with berries or honey at first.

From one mother: *"When I was introducing my children to fresh vegetables, I started cooking them with lots of butter and cheese to make them taste really good. Then I slowly reduced the amounts of butter and cheese. Gradually over time the veggies were served* *without the added taste enhancers. My children loved them and to this day they all love vegetables — both cooked and raw."*

SHAPE, DON'T CONTROL

There is a difference between these two concepts. In fact, studies have shown that when parents try to overcontrol their children's eating habits, it usually backfires. Overcontrolled children are more likely to become overfat and undernourished on fake food. Think of shaping versus control like tending a garden. You can't control the color of the flower or the time of the year it blooms,

---

BEWARE OF FOOD SABOTEURS

Day-care providers, babysitters, nannies, grandparents, even some nutrition-unsavvy teachers, can sabotage the healthy nutritional habits you've tried to instill in your child. One mother told me: "When my son went from two to three years of age, he gained ten pounds. My babysitter was giving him snack packs of Oreos and peanut butter sandwich crackers. Once I found out what had caused the sudden weight gain, I cut him back to the nutritious food he was used to. He went back to a normal weight gain."

Sometimes it's easy for your caregivers to reach for junk food as an easy pacifier, for example during a tantrum. But this only reinforces undesirable behavior, since the child learns that if he throws a tantrum, he gets a junk cookie. If you don't have junk food in your house, the babysitter won't be able to feed it to your children. Leave healthy and creatively prepared foods around the house so that your subs get the message: This is what you want your kids to eat.

but you can feed the soil and prune the plant so it blossoms more beautifully. That's shaping.

Avoid the "food Nazi" perception. Too many restrictions and too many food rules can backfire. And no food threats, please! "You can't watch TV until after you've eaten your carrots" is more likely, research shows, to cause the child to dislike carrots. On the other hand, seat a child at a table with a bunch of other carrot eaters and he is likely to eat carrots. Food researchers call these *positive and negative associations.*

Nutritional studies all come to the same conclusion: In homes where parents try to control their children's diets and impose lots of unrealistic restrictions, those children tend to grow up eating more unhealthy foods. But children who grow up in a real-food home with the "we principle" and healthy parental modeling tend to follow their parents' eating habits. *Parental modeling is more effective than parental control.*

It's okay, however, to set some rules in meal habits, such as "Eat your veggies before dessert" and "Grow foods before fun foods."

MAKE MEALS MORE FUN

As you gradually wean your child from fake foods to real foods, make mealtimes more exciting. Add more fun to the real foods so that your child will be so captivated by the new way of eating that he'll overlook the fact that he's eating different foods with different tastes. Your child will then associate real foods with fun eating. Make edible art. Children are more likely to eat what they create. Here are some ideas:

- *Whimsical waffles.* As you switch from enriched white to 100 percent whole-grain waffles, dress up the real-food waffles with happy faces made with fruit cut-outs: kiwi eyes, blue-berries for hair, and a strawberry nose. Your child will be so distracted by the creative happy face that he won't even no-tice you sneaked in a good-grain switch.

- *Perked-up pasta.* Going whole grain is more challenging when it comes to pasta. Make the sauce even more tasty. Make funny faces with olives and veggies on top of the sauce. Your children will be so sidetracked by the sauce, they will forget the "healthier" pasta underneath.

- *Pretty pizzas.* Spread tomato sauce on whole wheat pita bread or whole wheat English muffins. Make a face with slices of cheese, olives, strips of bell peppers, and chunks of tuna. Heat it in the oven until the cheese starts to melt.

- *Smiley sandwiches.* Cut out whole wheat sandwiches with cookie cutters and decorate them with pieces of vegetables, such as olive eyes, grated carrot curls, and a cherry tomato nose on top of hummus.

- *Cute cookies.* If your child is a cookie maker, gradually change from white flour to 100 percent whole wheat flour and use raisins, dates, or honey as a sweetener. Make the cookies so cute that your children are distracted and overlook the fact that the cookies are less sweet than the cookies they were previously used to.

- *Colorful caterpillars.* Put cut-up fruits and veggies on skew-ers. Serve with a yogurt dip.

- *Pretty pancakes.* Make faces on 100 percent whole wheat pan-cakes: banana slices and a raisin pupil for the eyes, a sliver of cantaloupe for the mouth, a yogurt beard, guacamole eyebrows, and a strawberry nose.

Remember, as you go "pure," you have to go more creative.

MAKE "HAPPY MEALS"

No, not the fast-food type. Studies show that children are more likely to accept a new food and healthy food in the context of a pleasant experience rather than one filled with restrictions and rewards. Enjoy happy talk at happy meals. Tell funny stories to make your child laugh — between bites. Enjoying this new way of relating at mealtimes will help your child accept this new way of real-food eating.

At our family meals, we try for only happy talk. Reserve the appetite-killers for non-mealtimes. At mealtimes we observe the KISMIF principle: Keep it simple, make it fun.

From one mother: *"We joke with our kids that we can see their muscles getting bigger whenever they eat some good protein foods. Our motto is 'Try something once.' Green Eggs and Ham has been a favorite book in our house, so I say, 'Sam would be so proud of you if you just tried it once!' If my five-year-old doesn't finish her breakfast, I tell her she can come back later when she gets hungry for a snack or a 'second breakfast.' Quite often she comes back to the table ten minutes later to finish it up. I think that using each time we eat as a possibility for a 'mini meal' keeps kids from being gluttonous."*

Model eating real foods. I can't overemphasize the importance of the "we principle" in marketing real food to children. What children see you do and what goes into your mouth make more of an impression than what you say. You're hungry, you reach for an apple. Next time your child says, "I'm hungry," simply point to the bowl of fruit on the counter and let him self-select. Your child will then replay that stored image in his mind of Mommy eating an apple when she's hungry. When children see the rest of the family eating real food, it makes a lasting impression. He thinks, "I guess this is what people are supposed to eat." Surround your child with pictures of real food.

MAKE REAL FOODS PART OF REAL LIFE

When you eat out, choose restaurants that have a salad bar. Hang out at farmers markets. Go real-food picking at farms. Join produce co-ops. When children grow up in the world of real food, that becomes *their* real world.

What doesn't work is to buy junk food, put it in the fridge or pantry, and then tell your children they can't eat it. What's wrong with this picture? Your child thinks, and rightly so, "If my parents buy it and stock it, it must be okay to eat." This is another example of where food restrictions will backfire. If there is a bag of junk chips sitting in the pantry and you tell your child, "You can't eat them," with the lame excuse, "They aren't good for you," that only increases the child's desire to eat the "forbidden food." Out of sight is out of mind. Have only real foods in your house.

Healthy birthday to you! Next time you're having a birthday party, call all the other parents ahead of time and suggest a real-food party. During this party, serve only real foods, but present them in an extra fun way. Bake a homemade cake. Introduce some new foods. When the other children are hungry, for example, after playing, they'll eat just about anything you serve. When your child sees other kids eating new foods, this bit of peer pressure should pay off, and he will likely copy them.

SCIENCE SAYS: CHILDREN TEND TO EAT WHAT THEY SEE OTHER CHILDREN EAT.

In 2003, food researchers from the University of Wales studied four hundred children ages four to eleven. Over a sixteen-day span, these children watched six video adventures called *The Food Dudes,* featuring heroic peers who enjoyed eating fruits and veggies. During and following the video-watching days, consumption of the foods they had seen their peers eating in the videos went way up. There were two reasons for this: (1) The "we principle" — children got the message that real kids eat real food; and (2) There were rewards. The kids eating real food were shown to have bigger muscles and to be able to run faster, and the kids concluded that food improved their sports performance.

Read what our daughter Hayden did for a healthy birthday party for our four-year-old granddaughter Ashton:

"The health-conscious part of me dreads kids' birthday parties, which come at least a couple of times a month. It is not so much the token cake and ice cream that I mind but the hot dogs, chips, candy, soda, punch, and goody bag that wreak havoc in my dear child's body. Is this excess really necessary? I would love to propose another way to celebrate each year of precious life. Let me explain by describing my daughter Ashton's birthday party. The guests and their parents got to snack on fresh veggies with guacamole and hummus, a big bowl of red grapes, and some trail mix. They sipped water and 100 percent juice. For lunch we had a fun activity of making 'pretty pizzas.' Everyone got their own whole wheat English muffin or whole wheat pita. On top they spread their own sauce and sprinkled their own cheese.

"Then they got to be creative, decorating their pizza with a variety of veggies. They used shredded carrots as hair, kidney beans as eyes, olives as noses, and red bell pepper strips for the lips. Some people made landscapes or race cars. Then we baked the pizzas at 400° for about ten minutes. The kids and parents had a blast eating their own creations while getting a wonderful amount of nutrients. For the cake, Ashton and I made a simple yellow cake. We topped it with beautiful strawberries and homemade whipped cream. Instead of mounds of frosting, I stuck in fun candles and a plastic 'Happy Birthday' sign. It was a hit! People left feeling treated to something special but without the sugar crash that most parents dread. Hey, moms, let's band together and create parties that will build our kiddos up."

TWENTY WAYS TO INTRODUCE NEW FOODS TO PICKY EATERS

The most common complaints we get from parents who are trying to "go pure" and feed their children grow foods are "My child is such a picky eater" and "My kids just have trouble accepting new foods." Here are twenty time-tested tricks from the Sears family kitchen and from parents in our pediatric practice:

1. Nibble it. Offer kids a "nibble tray." Use an ice-cube tray, muffin tin, or other compartmentalized dish and put bite-size portions of nutritious food in each section. Call the foods in the nibble tray child-friendly names such as:

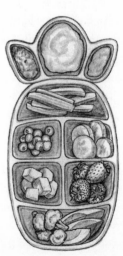

- apple moons (peeled apple slices, with or without peanut butter)
- avocado boats (quarter an avocado sliced lengthwise)

Dr. Sears' Nibble Tray™

- banana wheels
- broccoli trees (steamed broccoli florets)
- cheese "blocks"; tofu "blocks"
- egg canoes (hard-boiled egg wedges)
- little O's (O-shaped cereal)
- sticks (cooked carrots or whole wheat bread)

2. Dip it. Children like to dip and dunk. Dipping less favored foods, especially veggies, in a favorite dip is a sure winner. Using a dipping bowl, try these dips:

- cheese sauce
- chickpea puree (hummus)
- cottage cheese
- guacamole (with or without spices)
- nut butters
- nutritious salad dressing
- pureed fruit or cooked vegetables
- refried beans
- tofu puree
- yogurt (plain or flavored with fruit concentrate)

3. Spread it. Young children liike spreading and smearing. Let them smear nutritious spreads (avocado, cheese, meat pâté, peanut butter, hummus, vegetable sauce, pear or other fruit concentrates) on crackers, bagels, toast, or rice cakes.

4. Top it. Toddlers and older children are into toppings. Putting familiar and nutritious favorites on top of new and less desirable foods is a way to broaden the finicky toddler's menu. Toppings include melted cheese, yogurt, cream cheese, guacamole, pear concentrate, tomato sauce, meat sauce, applesauce, and peanut butter.

5. Sip it. If your child would rather drink than eat, no problem. Make a nutritious fruit-and-yogurt smoothie. Smoothies are a Mommy favorite for sneaking in new grow foods. You can sneak a lot of nutritious foods into a smoothie that you wouldn't normally be able to get your toddler to eat. After your child gets used to enjoying a certain smoothie mixture, slip in a new food once or twice a week, such as spinach or tofu. Your child won't notice the tofu is in there, since it does not change the smoothie taste very much. Go slowly with the spinach, however. It's more detectable by color and taste. (For add-in suggestions, see page 139.)

From one mother: *"As long as we add a tablespoon of peanut butter, the kids can't taste the broccoli and spinach we put in the smoothie. If we run out of peanut butter, it tastes really 'green' and the kids won't eat it. We have found that peanut butter is the ultimate camouflage. Also, if you add lots of berries, the smoothie remains purple, even with all the veggies in it."*

---

6. Bite it. Try the "two-bites test." Don't expect love at first bite. Say, "Take two bites . . . and you can have more if you want . . . or you can try it another time." Don't say, "if you don't like it." Planting negative thoughts in a child's suspicious mind is a setup for a food refusal.

From one mother: *"We use the one-bite-for-each-year-of-age trick. For a three-year-old, that means three bites of chicken, three bites of rice, three bites of veggies."*

---

7. Sneak it. Here are some fun ways to sneak grow foods and new foods into picky eaters. Cut nutritious veggies into small pieces and put them *under* a proven favorite food, such as cheese. Hide the salmon between the tomato sauce and the pasta. Sprinkle sprouts between the peanut butter and jam on a whole wheat

PB&J sandwich. The seven most versatile foods into which to sneak new foods are:

1. Avocado. Great guacamole! Dip any food into it.

2. Beans. Mash them and dip into them.

3. Low-fat cheese. Make sauces, dips, and toppings with the cheese.

4. Nut butters. Spreads and dips camouflage what's underneath.

5. Mashed potatoes. Put a piece of salmon on top or underneath.

6. Yams. Whip them up and consider mashing in some yogurt, flaxseed oil, or cooked veggies, such as lentils. A yam-and-cheese quesadilla is yummy.

7. Yogurt. Sneak in berries and ground flaxseeds.

From one mother: "When my toddler went through a stage of food refusals, for example eating only pancakes for breakfast, I just smiled and added eggs instead of water and used 100 percent whole-grain pancake mix. At least I knew he was getting some protein for breakfast. Then I began adding other things to the pancakes, such as three or four bittersweet chocolate chips instead of syrup. I even started making the pancakes with peanut butter and put jelly without added sweetener on them."

---

8. Grind it. For children under four, grind chokable foods such as flaxseeds and sunflower seeds, and sprinkle them onto oatmeal or into smoothies or salads.

SPECIAL SPRINKLES

Kids love sprinkles. They make food fun besides being a creative way to sneak in healthy nutrients and shape young tastes. Here are the ones we use in our family:

- cinnamon
- coconut
- dark chocolate flakes
- flaxseed meal
- nuts, finely chopped

---

9. Dice it. Dice raw, leafy greens such as spinach, chard, and kale (often the least favorite, but the most nutritious) and cook them into spaghetti sauce, bury them in mashed potatoes, or hide them in a smoothie.

10. Spice it up. Add some herbs and spices to your child's life. Not only do they make foods more flavorful, but new research is showing that they sneak in lots of health benefits, such as helping to regulate blood sugar and acting as natural anticancer nutrients and anti-inflammatories. One of our granddaughters will try any new food if we sprinkle cinnamon on it. Try these herbs and spices:

- cinnamon
- ginger
- rosemary
- turmeric

11. Squeeze it. Squeeze a cut lime and sprinkle it over salads. This not only gives the veggies a more tangy taste but also adds some vitamin C and acidity that helps some of the nutrients from the veggies be more easily digested.

12. Sweeten it. Children are born with a sweet tooth (mother's milk is very sweet). To wean them off the taste of artificial sweeteners, gradually decrease the fake sweeteners and add instead honey, guava nectar, fruit concentrates, mashed fruits (such as blueberries and strawberries), and cinnamon.

13. Cook it. Enjoy some fun mother-child kitchen time, and let your child help you cook. Just as children are more likely to eat what they have grown, they are more likely to eat what they helped prepare and cook. Capitalize on the "I do it myself" stage from two to four years old. Mashing potatoes is a sure winner. In fact, any food mashed is more likely to make it into a child's mouth. Make whole wheat oatmeal cookies. Teach your child how to spread the peanut butter and fruit juice–sweetened jelly on whole wheat bread. Show your child how to use cookie cutters to create edible designs out of foods she likes, such as whole wheat bread, thin meat slices, or cooked lasagna noodles. Give your little assistant fun jobs, such as washing and tearing lettuce, scrubbing potatoes, and stirring batter. Put pancake batter in a squeeze bottle and guide her hands as she squeezes the batter on the griddle in fun shapes, such as hearts, numbers, or even her name.

The more you involve children in the food preparation, the more likely they are to try it and to enjoy it.

14. Organize it. Give your child his own shelf space in the refrigerator. Reserve a low shelf for all of your child's favorite nutritious foods and drinks. Nibbling on nutritious foods during the day mellows a child's erratic moods by encouraging him to eat when he's hungry. Giving your children a place of their own allows you to stock the shelf, and when they say, "Mom, I'm hungry," you can say, "Help yourself to your shelf."

15. Shrink it. Keep servings small. Ever wonder why toddlers seldom clean their plates? A toddler's tummy is about the size of his fist. As a graphic exercise, place your toddler's fist next to the usual plateful of food you offer him. You can see the mismatch and understand why your child seldom finishes every bite on his plate. Grazing on frequent minimeals throughout the day is more in keeping with a toddler's temperament and tummy size. Think quality, not quantity.

16. Dilute it. Children love fruit juice, but too much is too many sweet calories. The American Academy of Pediatrics recommends limiting fruit juice to eight ounces a day. Dilute fruit juice with half water or sparkling water. Or sneak in a bit of veggie juice (try carrot juice or ground greens juice, available at many nutrition stores and Trader Joe's) and gradually increase the amount of veggie juice as you decrease the concentrations of fruit juice.

17. Time it. Studies show that children are most likely to try new foods when they are the most hungry.

18. Share it. Let peer pressure work to your advantage. Try group feeding. Invite over a same-age toddler who likes to eat nutritious foods and let your child catch the spirit. Or have a mini "dinner for two." Offer the new foods: "Mommy takes a bite. . . . Billy takes a bite." Put the food on your plate. Capitalize on the copycat stage by setting your child on your lap and putting the new food on your plate. Proceed with enjoying the meal and watch your child start picking the new food off your plate. In our family we have noticed that our toddlers will try more foods while sitting on our laps and eating off our plates.

19. Exaggerate it. Children love to play copycat. When offering your child a new food or one that has been previously refused, let your child see you eating it yourself. As you're chomping on the broccoli floret, make a happy face. Smile (it's okay to let a few greens show through your teeth) and say, "Yum, yum!" Your child is likely to want to grab a piece of broccoli off your plate and copy you.

From one mother: *"We have a high chair that pulls right up to the table, with no plastic tray in front. Our daughter sat at the table with us from the time she was five and a half months. We love good food, and she seems to just copy us. I really didn't think she would like asparagus, but my husband grilled a bunch of veggies for me, and I fed them to her as well. I feed her new stuff without flinching or indicating anything is new. We just eat and treat her like a person who has a developed palate like us."*

20. Grow it. Plant a garden together. Kids are likely to eat what they help grow. They are so proud of their accomplishments that they can't wait to taste what they grew.

From one mother: *"We grow cherry tomato plants and encourage our kids to pick and eat them anytime."*

Make every calorie count. Offer your child nutrient-dense foods. Kid favorites include salmon, avocado, cheese, eggs, sweet potatoes, nut butters, and yogurt. Count on inconsistency. Children may eat a food one day and then not touch it the next. As a parent in our practice said, "The only thing consistent about feeding children is inconsistency." Be flexible and don't take it personally. Remember, your responsibility is to buy the right food, prepare it nutritiously, and serve it creatively. The rest is up to your child.

6

Step 3: Begin the Day with a Brainy Breakfast

As we've discussed, the brain above all other organs is affected for better or worse by what we eat. If a child starts school with junk food in the brain, you get junk learning and junk behavior. It's as simple as that! This is especially true when you break a fast. Unlike other organs, the brain does not store glucose. The child has just gone eight to ten hours without food, and the reserve tank is nearly empty. Just as you wouldn't drive your car to work on an empty tank, you shouldn't drive the brain to school without fuel.

FOUR BENEFITS OF A BRAINY BREAKFAST

Here's how a brainy breakfast helps break the epidemic of NDD:

1. Breakfast eaters are smarter students. One of the best ways to prevent a teacher from labeling your child with a school-related D such as ADD is to begin his day with smart food. Breakfast builds smarter brains. Studies show that compared with breakfast skippers and junk-food-breakfast eaters, children who begin the day with a brainy breakfast enjoy:

- higher grades
- better attention and participation in class
- higher reading and math scores
- improved memory, especially on complex tasks
- fewer Ds: ADD, ADHD, OCD, and *d*epression

2. Breakfast eaters are healthier students. Studies reveal that kids who begin the day with a brainy breakfast miss fewer days of school because of sickness. This is most likely due to their healthier immune systems. If you start the day off with a body and brain full of germ-fighting phytos, you get sick less often. Makes sense!

3. Breakfast eaters tend to be leaner. Lean kids suffer fewer illnesses and sports injuries than do overfat children. By a biochemical quirk called *front loading,* kids who begin the day with adequate nutrition tend to need fewer calories the rest of the day. Breakfast skippers or junk-breakfast eaters, on the other hand, often compensate by overeating the rest of the day.

4. Breakfast eaters eat better all day. Studies also show that breakfast sets the nutritional habits for that day. Begin the day with a healthy breakfast and a "smart switch" seems to turn on that prompts the child to crave healthy food throughout the day. Food researchers fed one group of kids a junk-food breakfast and another group a brainy breakfast. These two groups automatically chose either junk food or real food from the school lunch offerings according to what they ate for breakfast.

A TALE OF TWO BREAKFAST EATERS

To appreciate how a brainy breakfast benefits school performance and learning, let's get into the brains of two schoolchildren. Johnny is a habitual breakfast skipper or junk-breakfast eater, and Brenda begins the day with a brainy breakfast. Notice how each behaves and learns.

Brenda Brainy Breakfast

Brenda got up in the morning after a restful night's sleep and sat down to a bowl of warm oatmeal that had slowly cooked in a Crock Pot overnight. On top of her steel-cut Irish oatmeal, Brenda's mother sprinkled blueberries and Greek yogurt. This was accompanied by a glass of organic milk. Off to school Brenda went, feeling satisfied but not too full. When she entered the classroom, her body and brain were in biochemical balance.

When school began, Brenda's brain was primed to learn. The high-protein breakfast perked up the learning and alertness neurotransmitters, dopamine and norepinephrine. Proteins and fiber-filled carbs triggered the calming neurohormone serotonin. Her brain was both alert and settled. The digestion in her gut brain was calm because of the friendly foods in it, so her gut didn't steal blood from her brain.

When her carbo-craving brain said, "I need sugar," the gut brain obliged by slowly releasing just the right amount into her blood. Because of this, her insulin remained stable — not too high, not too low. Because her insulin, the master conductor in the biochemical orchestra of hormones in her body, stayed stable, her brain was in hormonal harmony. She was alert, calm, ready to learn.

By ten o'clock her brain began to use up her breakfast fuel. Her mother had advised her not to wait until she got hungry to eat, so at break, she nibbled on a bag of nuts. Her brain stayed in biochemical balance. She behaved well and learned. All day she was around kids who were coughing, but she didn't get sick. Her body was full of germ-fighting phytos.

Because Brenda started the day with grow foods, her body was programmed to crave similar foods for the rest of the day. She was biochemically "addicted" to the good feelings in both her gut brain and her head brain.

Because she began the day in biochemical balance, her food-craving hormones were not erratic, so she didn't binge or overeat for the rest of the day. As a result, instead of being overfat, she stayed lean, and this helped her stay in biochemical balance. Biochemically balanced Brenda truly had a head start.

Johnny Junk Breakfast

Johnny awoke after a restless night's sleep. After wolfing down a Pop-Tart and a glass of Hi-C punch, he rushed off to school, his body in biochemical imbalance. Without the protein to perk up his brain, his alertness neurohormones were low. Without the proteins and good carbs to trigger calming neurohormones, his brain was unsettled. His mind drifted from what the teacher was teaching the class. His eyes wandered from the blackboard to the window as he thought about how he'd rather be outside running than inside learning.

By nine thirty he was hungry. The junk carbs had rushed into his blood so fast that they were all used up. His insulin, which was previously too high to handle the early sugar rush, had triggered all sorts of biochemical mischief. When hunger came, he was already hypoglycemic (low in blood sugar) and out of balance, and his mind was out the window. The combination of hunger and low blood sugar triggered stress hormones. The body hates to be hungry and out of fuel, so it releases the stress hormone cortisol to squeeze stored sugar out of the liver and rush it to the brain.

Now Johnny was even more out of biochemical balance. His alertness hormones never got going, nor did his calming hormones. His bloodstream was a mixed-up biochemical soup. His stress hormones surged. His body fidgeted and his mind wandered. "He must be another one of those kids with ADD," his teacher concluded.

"He needs to be drugged for his Ds," Johnny's teacher told his parents. The hurried D doctor agreed. Now Johnny begins the day with his brain out of biochemical balance from NDD and further out of balance from another D — drugs.

Because Johnny begins the day with junk food, his body is programmed to eat junk food the rest of the day. So his NDD lasts the rest of the day — and night. By the time Johnny goes to bed, the effect of the drug is supposed to wear off so that he can sleep restfully, but it doesn't. A brain that is out of biochemical balance during the day becomes a brain out of balance at night. So Johnny wakens already out of biochemical balance and then gets more out of biochemical balance after eating a junk-food breakfast, and the sick cycle of Ds continues.

Who do you want your child to be like, Brenda Brainy Breakfast or Johnny Junk Breakfast?

FOUR STEPS TO SERVING A BRAINY BREAKFAST

Now that you're convinced that you want your family to begin the day with a brainy breakfast, here's how to make it happen.

1. Tell your children why a brainy breakfast is better. Announce the change to your children and explain why you are doing it. Either read the Tale of Two Breakfast Eaters, above, to them or put it in your own words. Remember our motto: Food needs to be fun. Emphasize how much more fun they'll have at school if their brains are able to focus better and their bodies have more energy. Tell them they'll better enjoy the time spent in the classroom and the after-school activities.

Children are performance-oriented. Feed them the message that a brainy breakfast leads to a happier day. If possible, sit down and enjoy breakfast with your children so you can model the importance of the meal. Tell them you are eating a brainy breakfast so that you can have a happier and smarter day at work, or equate what you eat for breakfast with how your day is going to go in whatever way works best.

Encourage your children to make a list of breakfast grow foods when you shop. Give them choices the night before of what they might want for breakfast so there are no surprises or food hassles in the morning.

2. Have a happy meal. Remember your goal is to help your children's brains begin the day in biochemical balance. As you previously learned, stress hormones cause the brain to be out of balance. Save upsetting criticisms or corrections ("You need to do better at math . . .") for another time of the day. A happy breakfast sends your children off to school with a brain full of happy hormones.

3. Insist on the best ingredients. The two top grow ingredients for the brain are proteins and omega-3 fats. Yet, the standard American diet (SAD) is sadly deficient in these nutrients for breakfast. A brainy breakfast should include:

- *proteins* to perk up the brain: eggs, yogurt, whole grains, and nut butters
- *phytos* to boost the immune system: colorful fruits and veggies
- *fiber-filled carbs* to provide a steady supply of fuel
- healthy *fats,* such as omega-3s, to build brain tissue
- mindful *minerals,* such as calcium and iron, to boost brain biochemistry

---

WET THE APPETITE!

Morning dehydration from overnight dryness can cause a queasy stomach and dampen the appetite.

From one mother: "*I have my child drink a glass of water as soon as she gets out of bed. This seems to settle her stomach and perk up her appetite for breakfast.*"

Why does your child need a high-protein and good-carbs breakfast? Proteins perk up the brain by feeding neurochemicals that foster focusing and learning. Studies show that children who eat a high-protein breakfast score better on attention tests than kids who skip breakfast or eat junk-food breakfasts. Carbs feed the neurochemicals that also calm the brain. A brainy breakfast needs to be high in perky proteins and medium in calming carbs. A high-carb, low-protein breakfast (the standard American breakfast) has the opposite effect, slowing down brain activity rather than priming the brain for learning. While a high-carb meal usually makes adults sleepy, it can make children either sleepy or hyper.

Here's why carbs make you sleepy. Proteins contain two brainy amino acids: *tyrosine,* which feeds the focusing neurotransmitters, and *tryptophan,* which feeds serotonin, the calming and sleep-inducing neurohormone. When these two protein parts enter the brain, they need some direction to tell it whether to perk up or to go to sleep. Insulin is the traffic cop here. If the breakfast is high-carb, high insulin results. High insulin prefers to usher the tryptophan into the brain rather than the tyrosine. That's why you feel like taking a siesta after a high-carb lunch. A high-protein breakfast, on the other hand, perks up the alertness neurotransmitters. You want your child to be calm, alert, and focused.

It's interesting that proteins, especially those in the grow foods listed on page 99, have the perfect balance of the alertness and calming amino acids. In most grow foods there are more perking-up amino acids than calming ones, which is exactly what you want at school: alertness and calmness, but not sleepiness. On the other hand, the evening meal, especially dessert, can be primarily carbs, which stimulate the calming and sleepy hormones more than the perking-up ones — just what you want before bed, but not before school.

4. Enjoy twelve brainy breakfast ideas. Try to incorporate into your child's breakfast a mix of as many of these five foods as possible: eggs, yogurt, fruit, whole grains, and omega 3s.

- apple slices with peanut butter and yogurt
- Dr. Bill's School-Ade Smoothie for a breakfast on the run (see recipe, page 182).
- egg in the hole: egg in the middle of a slice of whole wheat toast, orange juice, fruit
- french toast topped with berries, side of yogurt
- "grow-food glass": Take an 8- to 10-ounce glass and fill half of it with yogurt. Then add a layer of whole-grain granola cereal and chopped fruits, such as apples and berries. Top it off with ground flaxseeds, a drizzle of honey, and slivered almonds. You can prepare this parfait the night before and store it in the refrigerator. (See recipe, page 185.)
- oatmeal, organic yogurt, blueberries
- omega-3 supplement (e.g., Brainy Kidz; see dosage, page 167)
- peanut butter on whole wheat toast topped with bananas or berries, glass of milk
- veggie omelet, homemade bran muffin, fruit

- whole-grain granola cereal, yogurt, and berries
- whole-grain waffles or pancakes topped with berries and yogurt, glass of milk
- zucchini pancakes topped with berries

WHY SMOOTHIES ARE SMART

I recommend smoothies often in my medical practice. They're a smart choice for many reasons.

Smoothies are great camouflage. Smoothies are an easy way to sneak in nutritious "grow foods" that you want your children to develop a taste for but that they won't eat, such as veggies, tofu, flaxseed meal, flax oil, or fish oil.

Smoothies provide nourishment easily for sick kids. Smoothies are super when children are too sick to eat but are willing to drink. Since food refusals often accompany childhood illnesses, in my pediatric practice I call smoothies the sipping solution to prevent dehydration and undernourishment while a child is recovering from an illness.

Smoothies promote good digestion. Smoothies soften bowel movements and are a very effective treatment for the common condition of childhood constipation. The high fiber in the fruit and ground grains, such as wheat germ and flaxseed meal and the flaxseed oil, are some of nature's best laxatives.

Smoothies can shape the kids' tastes. Smoothies are a fun way to gradually shape or reshape children's tastes toward eating more grow foods and fewer junk foods. By adding more of one food and less of another, you can gradually reshape tastes in the right direction, often without kids even realizing it.

From one mother: "*To get him to drink smoothies, I call them whatever he's into. This week he is devouring his 'dinosaur drink.'*"

Dr. Bill's best smoothie ingredients. Use these base ingredients:

- ground flaxseeds
- fruits: blueberries, strawberries, mango, papaya, pineapple, banana, kiwi
- juice (pomegranate, carrot, veggie juice, etc.) or organic milk
- organic yogurt

Use varying amounts of the following "special add-ins":

- cinnamon
- dates
- honey (usually the cinnamon, raisins, or dates in addition to the fruits will provide enough sweetness)
- multivitamin/multimineral protein powder
- omega-3 supplement, such as fish oil
- peanut butter
- raisins
- spinach leaves
- tofu
- wheat germ
- whey protein powder

Make a smiley straw. Make a smiley face on a Post-it and punch it over the straw in the smoothie bottle. Your children will notice your happy message every time they drink.

From one mother: "*I freeze smoothie leftovers into homemade smoothie pops.*"

7

Step 4: Raise a Grazer

One of the most healthful lifelong eating habits you can teach your children is Dr. Bill's rule of two's:

- Eat *twice* as often.
- Eat *half* as much.
- Chew for *twice* as long.

WHY GRAZING IS GOOD FOR KIDS

That tiny tummy, about the size of the child's fist, has been used to grazing since infancy. As toddlers are natural dippers and nibblers, schoolchildren prefer to become grazers. Grazing on frequent minimeals rather than gorging on fewer bigger meals is not only the way children would naturally choose to eat, it is one of the best ways to prevent NDD. Here's why.

Grazing is good for the brain. Remember our buzzwords for fueling the brain: *slow* and *steady*. Grazing on grow foods provides a slow and steady supply of fuel to the brain. And remember, the brain, unlike other organs, does not store food energy. So not only does it use more food energy but it "runs out of gas" more quickly. An unsteady fuel supply leads to unsteady moods and an unsteady ability to focus.

Back to brain biochemistry. Grazers have a stable level of insulin, that master hormone in your child's hormonal orchestra. When insulin is stable, the whole body and the brain are in biochemical balance — that is, primed to behave and learn. Stable blood sugar and blood insulin means stable focusing, behavior, and mood. This is why insulin is called the health hormone. Science says grazers tend to:

- be better able to focus and learn
- have steadier moods and behavior

In summary, grazing helps prevent NDD.

Grazers are less stressed. Insulin and the stress hormone cortisol have a sort of codependent relationship. If one is stable, so is the other. Since grazing stabilizes insulin, it also stabilizes stress hormones. As we discussed, unstable stress hormones lead to more unstable learning and behavior. In fact, many of the Ds are due not only to unstable insulin levels but also to unstable stress hormones. A fascinating study showed that people who kept their same diet but changed to more frequent minimeals had lower blood levels of insulin and cortisol. Isn't that what we want for our children, stable moods, stable behavior, and focused learning?

Grazing is good for the gut. Picture what happens when your little gorger hits the school cafeteria. He wolfs down a huge fatty meal. He doesn't chew very long because he wants to get out and play. This big bolus of partially digested food hits the stomach and intestines. The lower end of the intestinal tract is now forced to work overtime because the top end (chewing) didn't do its job. The gut says, "I've got too much work to do. I need some help!" So the gut-brain steals blood from the head-brain to help digestion. Excess undigested food causes reflux or heartburn, giving the child a generally uncomfortable gut feeling. Too much undigested food at the lower end causes constipation — another not-good gut feeling. By this time, he is expected to go back to class, sit still, and learn, when all he wants to do is sleep or recover from his midday binge. Remember, the intestines are the second-largest nervous system in the body (hence the term *gut brain*). So if the gut-brain is bothered, so is the head-brain.

Grazing is good for weight control. Grazers tend to be leaner than gorgers. Grazing promotes fat burning; gorging promotes fat storing. Let's go back to our master hormone, insulin, again. Insulin wears two hats. It helps the body burn calories and helps the body store calories. So if you eat more than the body needs, insulin tells the body to store the excess food as excess fat, usually around the middle.

Grazing keeps you from being an iBod. Remember, there is an epidemic of inflammatory Ds — all those "-itis" illnesses. (See the discussion of iBods on page 29.)

SCIENCE SAYS: OVERWEIGHT MAY LEAD TO UNDERACHIEVEMENT

The 2007 Early Childhood Longitudinal Study of thirteen thousand third-grade children showed that overfat children have significantly lower math and reading scores.

From one mother: *"I put little nibbles of nutritious foods within easy reach around the house. That way my daughter can nibble anytime she wants, especially when she's going through an independent stage. Because nutritious food is available to her all day long, we don't stress at mealtime if she doesn't finish her meal. And I don't stress about her being a picky eater, because I know she's picking good food. The relaxed attitude in our family really pays off."*

FIVE WAYS TO RAISE A GRAZER

Here's how to put my rule of two's into practice:

1. Start early. Toddlers are born nibblers and grazers. Our favorite Sears family toddler-feeding trick is to make a nibble tray, an ice-cube tray or muffin tin filled with nutritious nibbles. We give these nibbles child-friendly names like broccoli "trees," orange "wheels," tofu and cheese "blocks," and cooked carrot "sticks." Reserve a couple compartments for dips such as guacamole and yogurt. Put the nibble tray on the child's own shelf in the fridge or on a low table and let him self-serve throughout the day. By the end of the day, the tray will be empty and your child will be comfortably full — and without any food hassles. Once children get used to the good gut feelings from grazing and the bad gut feelings from gorging, this early habit is likely to last a lifetime. (For food suggestions for the nibble tray, see pages 122–123.)

2. Teach about the intestinal tract. Draw a picture of the intestinal tract. Begin with the mouth, and then draw the long tube of the esophagus entering a pouchlike stomach, followed by the long, windy tube of the intestines. Show your child what happens when too much food goes into the gut too fast: "The stomach gets big and uncomfortable and you get a tummyache. When too much food stays in the intestine, your poop gets big and hard like golf balls and it hurts when you go to the bathroom." Make this teachable moment as detailed as appropriate to your child's level of understanding. Your main message is *You eat well, you feel well.*

3. Play chew-chew. For another Show-and-Tell exercise, through your own chewing and by drawing a picture, show your child how chewing breaks up the food more at the top end. Chewing releases saliva, which contains digestive enzymes that break up the food even more and help it "slip down the slide" more comfortably. What you're teaching your child is a lifelong gut message: *The more you do to the food at the top end of the intestines, the less wear and tear on the bottom end.*

The rule of two's is especially helpful in one of the fastest-growing Ds among children: inflammatory bowel disease. The softer the food and the more quickly it passes through the intestines, the less wear and tear (inflammation) there is on the intestinal lining. Chewing also makes eating more enjoyable, allowing the taste and texture of the flavorful food to hang around in the mouth longer. Because chewing helps food be more satisfying, the child tends not to overeat, which is one of the reasons that grazers tend to be leaner. Mindless munching, on the other hand, chewing too little and too fast, is one of the most common causes of becoming overfat.

To help your child chew longer, encourage crunchy foods. Many kids like the sound and mouth feel of crunchiness, as cereal makers have known for a long time. It is one reason celery stalks filled with peanut butter or cheese puree are a very satisfying snack.

4. Have a "tummy talk." Teach your children to pay attention to their tummies. When the stomach says full, it's time to stop eating. This is another reason that chewing longer and eating more slowly helps. There is a delay of around fifteen to twenty minutes between when the stomach gets full and when it tells the brain to stop eating. If a child eats too fast, the stomach can get overfull long before the brain gets the message. To help your child chew longer, give him cute messages, such as, "Chew-chew times two" or "Chew twenty times." Have him count his chews a couple times so he gets used to chewing a set number of times.

5. Serve supersnacks. Have nutritious snacks readily available. Oftentimes adults get so busy they forget to offer snacks to children. The ideal snack should:

- have at least 5 grams of protein and 3 grams of fiber. Why? As you learned earlier, protein and fiber are fill-up foods, helping your child be satisfied longer and with less food.
- contain 100–200 calories
- be crunchy, requiring a lot of chewing
- be satisfying but not too filling
- contain any combination of the foods listed on page 148

SUPERSNACKS

Here's our list of snacks that we use in our family and recommend in our pediatric practice.

Nuts

Go nuts.* Nuts get my top vote for a supersnack for three reasons:

- They are nutrient-dense, packing a perfect blend of protein, healthy carbs, and healthy fats.

---

* For children over three to four years old, since nuts pose a choking hazard in toddlers.

- The high fiber content and protein–fat blend make nuts filling. This satiety quirk of nuts keeps children from overeating them.

- They are tasty. Kids love nuts and nut butters.

Food allergies. Around 6 percent of children have an allergy to some food, the most common of which are dairy, wheat, eggs, soy, shellfish, and nuts. Although population studies vary, it's estimated that about 1 percent of children is allergic to nuts. Even though this is a small percentage, a peanut allergy is the most serious of food allergies and can even be life-threatening. In a nut-by-nut case, peanuts are by far the most allergic nut (although peanuts are botanically a legume and not a nut) and lead to more severe allergies than tree nuts. While it used to be thought that peanut allergies were lifelong, the good news is that recent studies have shown that around 10 percent of children eventually outgrow their nut allergies. Another bit of good news is that children may be allergic to one nut but not to others. In fact, most people who are allergic to one or two types of nuts can find, by cautious trial and error, a nut they are not allergic to. Soy nuts are a safer alternative.

Make your own trail mix. Because each type of nut has specific nutrients, the best bang for your nut buck is to take a cupful of the following nuts and package your own trail mix:

- almonds: high in fiber, vitamin E, and calcium
- brazil nuts: high in the antioxidant selenium
- chestnuts: the lowest-fat nut
- hazelnuts: top nut for the sleep-inducing amino acid tryptophan
- macadamias: highest in good fat, which makes them a tasty favorite among chocolate-covered nuts

- peanuts: high in protein, folate, and niacin
- pecans: high in fiber, thiamin, and vitamin E
- pine nuts: high in zinc
- pistachios: top nut in vision-enhancing carotenoids, lutein, and zeaxanthin
- walnuts: highest in omega 3s

See the trail mix recipe on page 198.

Blend your own butters. Almond butter is a healthy alternative for children who are allergic to peanut butter, since these two nuts come from different families and therefore will not necessarily both cause allergies. Nut butters are a favorite for "sneakies." You can blend them in smoothies, spread them on bread or waffles, smear them on cookies, and dip fruits and vegetables in them. Nuts and nut butters are among the most healthy and versatile foods you can feed your children.

Bag your own nuts. Send your child off to school, play, or sports with a bag full of nuts. He can carry around his little nut bag and nibble whenever he is hungry. A palmful of nuts is also just what Mommy ordered to ward off those pre-meal hunger tantrums.

NUT BUTTER TIP: AVOID "BAD" BUTTER

Despite all the recommendations of top nutritionists, some popular peanut butter brands still contain hydrogenated oils, one of the bad words you learned about earlier. Check the label and avoid these brands.

SUPERSNACK LIST

Here's a list of good foods for grazing. These are supersnacks, ones that partner carbs with protein, fiber, and/or healthy fats. Your children will find lots to like on this list.

- apple slices dipped in peanut butter
- baby carrots dipped in hummus
- bean dip and veggie sticks
- blueberries in yogurt
- celery sticks with peanut butter
- cherry tomatoes with cheese cubes
- cottage cheese and fruit
- edamame (cooked soybeans)
- egg, hard-boiled
- fruit-and-yogurt smoothie
- fruit (any)
- oatmeal-raisin cookies, homemade
- Parmesan cheese melted on a slice of whole-grain bread
- pita bread spread with hummus
- popcorn (homemade air-popped)
- raw nuts or trail mix (a handful)
- rice cake with peanut butter and banana
- string cheese and a piece of fruit
- vegetables cut up with salsa and tortilla chips
- whole-grain cereal with yogurt
- whole-grain, preferably homemade, muffins

Other Nutritious Snacks

Go celery. Celery is another good snack because it's crunchy, it takes a long time to chew, and you can add nutritious fillings, such as peanut butter, hummus, and cheese.

Go yogurt. A top snack is a cup of plain yogurt with added fruit, such as blueberries and strawberries, and a dab of honey.

Go popcorn. Popcorn takes a while to eat and satisfies without overfilling the child. It is a great before-meal snack to tide over the hungry child.

Go eggs. Eggs are a perfect snack because for a mere 75 calories each they provide a rich source of protein, are filling, and have a high satiety factor. Eggs are versatile too: egg salad, deviled eggs, hard-boiled eggs, and "dip eggs," a poached or soft-boiled egg into which the child dips whole-wheat bread sticks.

Go fruits and veggies. Try edamame (cooked soybeans), an apple or orange, cherry tomatoes, bean dips with veggie sticks, apple slices dipped in peanut butter, and cut-up vegetables dipped in salsa.

Go cookies. Homemade oatmeal-raisin cookies or muffins are always hits. See the cookie recipe on page 201.

Edible balls. See the recipe for nutbutter balls, page 199. Pack two or three of these tasty balls in a small plastic bag. They make a perfect snack and between-meal treat.

Step 5: Encourage Healthy Eating When Out and at School

School-age children eat many of their meals outside Mom's kitchen, for example, at schools, in cars, at restaurants, and at friends' and relatives' homes. So how do you help your kids eat grow foods when someone else is serving the meals?

HOW TO HELP YOUR CHILD'S SCHOOL GET A PASSING GRADE IN NUTRITION

I served for four years as a member of a school board. One time at a meeting, I raised my hand and shocked the other members when I said, "I'm concerned about how easy it is for kids to get drugs at our school!" Now, please understand that this school worked hard to be drug-free. I went on: "Yes, in fact, right now for two dollars, I could walk fifty feet and buy drugs." They finally realized I was talking about the junk in the school vending machines. Folks forget that foods are drugs, good and bad.

From one mother: *"I spent the first five years raising pure children only to have them polluted when they got to school."*

Just as schools should model the family values taught at home, they should also model healthy eating habits. But it's in schools where most of the Ds are detected. Serving junk food at school presents a confusing message to a vulnerable child: "If school is supposed to teach me the right things, why do they serve junk food that Mommy says won't help me grow or learn?" Try these simple steps to keep your child pure at school:

Lobby for nutritious lunches. Academically, schools are only as good as the parents behind them. This is also true of the foods schools serve. You have both a right and an obligation to insist that the school not pollute your child. Here's an actual conversation I had with the principal at our child's school: "Why do we send our children to school?" I opened. He looked at me, rather puzzled, and I continued: "To give our children the tools to succeed in life, and teaching them what to eat is a valuable success tool." The principal got the point and agreed to make changes. To be sure this happened, a group of parents got together to visit the school cafeteria periodically during lunchtime and to check the contents of the vending machines, and we immediately complained if the junk food reappeared (which it occasionally did).

Lobby your school to begin the lunch line with a salad bar. This gives children the message that healthy food is crucial. It also gives children control over their choices.

Stephen, our teenage son with Down Syndrome, attends a special-needs class in a typical high school. His classmates have a variety of brain-wiring differences: cerebral palsy, autism, and other brain quirks. I imagined that a class full of quirky kids with quirky brains would certainly be fed brainy foods. Wrong! They were served the same junk food the typical kids got.

Schools are often not the problem. School cafeteria managers have told me that they have tried to serve healthy food, "but the children won't eat it." That's because healthy eating habits weren't modeled to children at home. The school should not be expected to reshape children's tastes. That has to be done by you.

Review the school menu with your child. If your child's school sends home a lunch menu, make this a teachable moment and review it with your child: "Let's see which one of these choices has the most grow foods." "Oops, that one has a bad word in it." "This one has lots of green-light foods." "This one looks like a smart school lunch." Circle the red-light foods and talk about them with your children. Then make an appointment with the school principal and cafeteria staff and show them where they are flunking lunch.

Pack your lunch. Remember the purpose of school food: to feed growing brains to help children learn and behave. If your school refuses to cooperate, brown-bag it. Here are ten nutritious and tasty suggestions:

- PB&J: peanut butter, almond butter, or soy nut butter, all-fruit jelly, 100 percent whole-wheat bread
- Fruit: apple, orange, a bunch of red grapes
- Veggies: cherry tomatoes; sliced red, yellow, and green peppers; raw broccoli florets; carrot sticks; celery sticks filled with peanut butter
- Trail mix. Make your own trail mix with a small bag of selected nuts, such as walnuts, almonds, pecans, and hazelnuts. Sprinkle in some raisins or dried cranberries and some sunflower seeds.
- A cup of plain Greek-style yogurt with a side of honey for sweetener
- Treats: peanut butter carob balls, homemade oatmeal-raisin cookies
- Hard-boiled egg

- Veggie wraps: whole wheat wrap or pita pocket with hummus and veggies; whole wheat pita pizza with tomato sauce and cheese
- Whole wheat tortilla burritos
- Container of guacamole with veggies (squeeze in a half lemon or lime juice to keep it fresh and colorful)

From one mother: "*I have a 'buy one time a week' policy for school lunches.*"

How many calories? While calorie-counting is less important if you pack a real-food lunch and a snack, here's a general guide: grades K–6: 600 calories, grades 7–12: 800 calories.

THE HEALTHIEST SCHOOL LUNCH BOX

The school lunch that is best for learning and behavior has four ingredients:

- proteins to perk up the brain
- grow carbs (partnered with protein and fiber) to fuel the brain
- right fats (e.g., nut butters, avocado)
- phytos to boost immunity

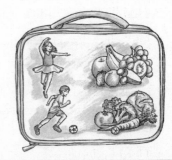

TRICKS TO CURB FOOD SWAPPING

You take great care to send your children off to day care, pre-school, or school with a pure lunch, only to have them polluted with fake food they trade with other kids. Kids will trade food, but here are some trading tricks you can use:

- Call a meeting of parents or make lots of phone calls. Have everyone agree to pack grow-food lunches, so at least if your child trades, he trades one grow food for another. Agree on packing snacks and lunches that have no "bad words" on the labels and that contain fiber-filled carbs and are high in protein. If your child is the only one with a healthy lunch, he may feel different, and children do not like to feel different.
- Pack little love notes that say, "Eat me, please don't trade me," or "I belong in your tummy. Please don't trade me."
- Ask the teacher to monitor the food trading.
- Make your child's lunch so good that he won't be tempted to trade. Remember, you're competing with colas. Kids will be kids, so they will trade if you don't provide them with tastier alternatives.
- When your child comes home, ask him what he ate for lunch. If he traded his lunch, ask him what foods he traded for. Discuss his food choices.

Personalize your child's school lunch.

- Add a little love note to the lunch box, saying, for example, "You've been blessed with a beautiful brain!" or "Mommy-made with love!"
- Label the food in terms that are more relevant to your child. For example, on the cherry tomato bag write, "Enjoy your little soccer balls."

(continued)

Personalize your child's school lunch, cont'd

- Put in a "smiley straw." Draw a smiley face and write a cute note on a Post-it and punch the straw through it.
- Let your child pick out a fun lunch box or snack containers.

PACK-A-SNACK TIPS

The magic word for best behavior and learning at school is *graze*. Studies show that consumption of a midmorning snack improves memory performance in schoolchildren. Ideally, your child should nibble on healthy midmorning and midafternoon snacks and have a light lunch. Here are some snack ideas:

- mixed nuts.* Make your own trail mix: nuts, raisins, dried fruit, sunflower seeds
- Popumz: a crunchy snack that packs 5 grams protein, 3 grams fiber, 32 milligrams omega 3s, and no "bad words" in each serving
- fruit: apple, orange, banana, pear
- homemade cookies: peanut butter, oatmeal-raisin
- celery sticks filled with nut butter
- edamame (cooked soybeans)
- legumes (e.g., kidney beans, chickpeas, lentils, and soybeans) have a very low glycemic index (meaning they have a steady release of carbs), which make them a perfect snack and lunch food.

(Also see supersnacks, page 148.)

---

* For children over three to four years old, since nuts pose a choking hazard for toddlers.

SIX TIPS FOR EATING HEALTHY WHEN NOT AT HOME

Eating out can be both novel and nutritious. Kids are more likely to try new foods when they are served in new places. But parents should do their homework to make eating out a healthy adventure.

1. Nibble on the way. Overhungry kids tend to overeat when eating out, especially at all-you-can-eat buffets. En route to the restaurant, encourage your child to eat a light snack.

2. Patronize "grow food" restaurants. Getting into an I-want-that, you-can't-have-that food fight robs your family of the fun of eating out. Frequent restaurants that don't hype junk food to kids. Grill the owner or waiter about the health quality of the food. Here are some sample questions to ask:

- Are your foods free of trans fats?
- Do you add chemical flavor-enhancers such as MSG?
- Do you use artificial colorings and sweeteners?

3. Can kids' menus. Kids' menus cause NDD. It's as simple as that. Tell your children the truth. Just because they are kids doesn't mean they should be served junk food. Be positive: "Guess what? You get to order from the grown-up menu!" Either ask for a smaller portion at a lower price or share an adult entrée between two children.

4. Eat salads first. If you're going to an all-you-can-eat restaurant, steer your kids to the salad bar first. If they fill up on salad, they are less likely to overeat.

5. Go international. Children are more likely to eat ethnic food if it's served in an ethnic restaurant. Let your children help choose the restaurant.

6. Grow foods before fun foods. In restaurants, the junkiest food is usually found in the desserts. Restaurant desserts are likely to contain all the bad words. So you have three choices: (1) let your children have whatever dessert they want provided they've eaten all the grow foods first; (2) let them choose a seminutritious dessert, such as fruit over ice cream rather than caramel sauce full of artificial sweeteners and colorings; or (3) treat them with a homemade pie or cake when they get home. To help them accept delaying their dessert gratification, say, "We're all full now. By the time we get home, our tummies will like having the dessert even more."

EATING AT FRIENDS' AND RELATIVES' HOMES

Many parents have the same complaints about the food at other people's homes as they do about the food at school. Try these tips to avoid having your child polluted at friends' and relatives' homes:

"Our doctor says he's allergic to . . ." I use this trick in my pediatric practice. If your child is going to have a prolonged visit at a friend's or relative's home where the nutrition is suspect, tell the food-making parents ahead of time: "Dr. Bill says that Amy is allergic to artificial food colorings and sweeteners, hydrogenated fats, high fructose corn syrup, and chemical flavor-enhancers, like MSG." Write these down and leave a list. As you learned in chapter 2, this is not a lie. I believe all children are allergic to these chemical additives — some show it now, while others will show it later. The word *allergies* gets people's attention, as they visualize a child having a wheezing fit after eating peanuts.

Tell the truth. If you are going through a family makeover to change your home into a pure one, tell the other people. Share with them that you are trying to wean your child off junk food and reshape her tastes toward healthy food. You might even dangle a motivating, "because they seem to bother her behavior so much." (The friend or grandparent doesn't want a misbehaving child in the home.) Elicit their help by offering, "Perhaps if Suzy sees that your family eats a lot of vegetables, she won't think I'm such a weird cook after all." A little peer pressure goes a long way. You may find that the other people like this idea as a way to get their own children to eat healthy foods: "Suzy is coming for dinner tonight, and I hear she loves vegetables, so we're going to make some special vegetables for her tonight."

Of course, a few of Grandmother's homemade chocolate chip cookies, while perhaps not being what the doctor ordered, are certainly what the doctor would eat. In fact, just about anything that Grandmother makes is a yellow-light treat food.

9

Step 6: Raise a Supermarket-Savvy Shopper

The supermarket is a giant nutritional classroom. Use it. Kids love it. While food shopping for most families is as exciting as a trip to a Laundromat, there are ways to make it fun.

Pre-shop. Tell your children, "We're going grow-food shopping." Encourage your child to help you make a list, adding her favorite grow foods, including, of course, a few treats. You might even compare your list with the traffic-light list on page 78 that you attached on your fridge (you did put our chart on your fridge, didn't you?). Be sure your shopping list contains mostly green-light grow foods, perhaps a few yellow-light foods, and no red-light foods.

Go directly to the grow foods. As you enter the supermarket, say to your child, "We only shop the *perimeter.* That's where the grow foods are." Quickly bypass the junk-food ads near the entrance and go directly to the produce section.

Go greens! Ask your child to grab some greens. Play Show-and-Tell. If she chooses a head of iceberg lettuce, here's a lettuce lesson: "Honey, we call that *see-through lettuce.* It's not a grow food.

> **Dr. Sears says:** Can the cartoon characters. If your child picks up a package of food with his favorite character on the front, it's a teachable moment: "Okay, Billy, you're a smart boy. What does Darth Vader know about grow foods that are good for you?"

Notice how pale it is? That's because it doesn't contain much grow food." Show her a head of romaine lettuce or spinach. "Notice you can't see through these greens. That's because they contain lots of grow foods. These are good-for-you greens."

From one mother: "Once a week we go to the farmers market together. That way she is exposed to all the wonderful fresh foods available, none of which come in shiny packages or with cartoon characters emblazoned on them."

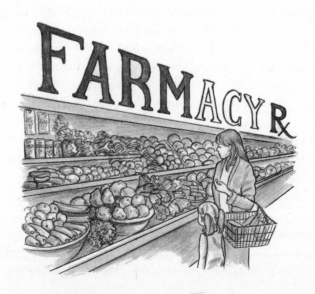

Go colors! Say, "Besides greens, let's select some colorful fruits and vegetables. Pick out two blues, three reds, three yellows, and two oranges. The deeper the color, the more grow foods it contains."

From one mother: *"She has her own canvas bag to fill with goodies she helps pick out."*

Grow foods first. For older children, impress upon them that grow foods keep them healthy. When your children see the shopping cart filling up first with produce, they get the message that these are the most important grow foods. As you continue around the perimeter, you select more grow foods, such as dairy products, eggs, lean meat, poultry, and fish. You're circling the supermarket, avoiding the interior as much as possible. If your child asks you about certain middle aisles, say: "Oh, that's where the red-light foods are. We just don't go there. Those aren't grow foods."

Eat grow breads. As you're shopping the perimeter, make a learning stop at the bread rack. Have your child pick up a loaf of white bread in one hand and a loaf of 100 percent whole wheat

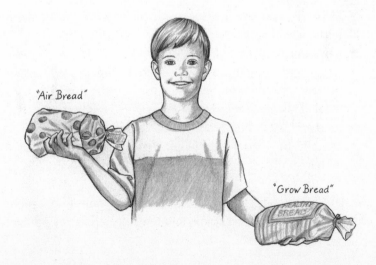

bread in the other. Ask her, "Do you feel any difference?" If you get an answer such as "Mommy, the white bread feels squishy," take that as a teachable moment and respond, "Do you want your muscles to feel squishy like the white bread or nice and firm like the whole wheat bread?" You want your children to learn that the foods they eat become the body they get. "Do you notice any other difference? Which one weighs more?" Your child will notice that the whole wheat loaf of bread is heavier. "That's because it contains more grow food," you say, adding, "We call white bread 'air bread' because it doesn't have as much grow food in it."

Try yummy yogurt. As you browse the yogurt section, more teachable moments pop up. It's a shame what they've done to this healthy green-light grow food. Most yogurts are now in the yellow-light category. A few deserve to be downgraded to the red-light category. Here's a good label lesson for your child. The "yummy yogurt" label has only two ingredients: milk and probiotics (acidophilus), and perhaps some added fruit. Teach your child three rules to picking yogurt. A grow-food yogurt:

- has only two ingredients: organic milk and probiotics (and perhaps added fruit)
- is organic (e.g., Stonyfield)
- has a higher protein-to-calorie ratio. Compare the grams of protein with the number of calories on the nutrition facts label. This generally means the yogurt contains more real food and fewer fillers.
- contains no "bad words": high fructose corn syrup or dyes with a number symbol, such as red #40

Go fish! Next comes a fishing lesson. Show your child a piece of wild salmon (firm, dark, pink, and few fatty streaks). Compare

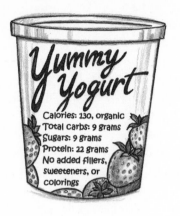
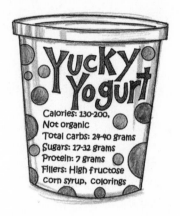

it with a piece of farm-raised salmon (soft, pale, and with fatty streaks). Then say, "The dark-colored, strong fish ate grow food and swam hard upstream. The pale, weak fish paddled in a pool all day and ate junk food. Which fish would you like your muscles to be like?"

Eat muscle meats. Peer into the meat counter and zoom onto a typical slab of sirloin steak. Ask your child what he sees. His response may be, "A lot of white stuff in the meat." Respond with, "That white stuff is fat, which makes the muscles weak and flabby. This muscle was taken from a steer that sat around and ate junk-food all day." Next take your child to a specialty market and have her compare the grain-fed, pen-raised, fatty piece of meat at the supermarket with a much leaner cut from grass-fed, free-range beef, which has a darker red color with fewer fatty streaks. Another teachable moment: "That piece of muscle came from an animal who ran and played outside a lot and ate healthy food." Ask your child, "Which muscle would you like to have?"

Go grains. After you've navigated the perimeter, cautiously venture into the cereal section. Play "I spy with my little eye . . . a bad word" (e.g., HFCS, hydrogenated, a number symbol). Lead your child to the "green-light cereals," which contain:

- *whole* wheat or other grains, not just wheat (the word *enriched* on a label is a clue that the bread is *not* whole wheat)
- at least 5 grams of protein per serving
- at least 3 grams of fiber per serving
- no more than 5 grams of added sugar
- no added artificial sweeteners, e.g., high fructose corn syrup, sucralose, aspartame
- no "bad words," e.g., red #40, hydrogenated oils, MSG
- bonus: added iron, calcium, zinc, vitamins, folate, DHA

Go for good snacks. Children enjoy snacks for good grazing. Instead of succumbing to the temptation of the junky snacks at the checkout counter, teach your child to look for grow-food snacks. Green-light snack or energy bars enjoy a similar nutrient composition to the green-light cereals above. Grow-food snacks should contain:

- at least 5 grams of protein and 3 grams of fiber per serving. (These two ingredients make the snack satisfying but not too filling.)
- a crunchy texture (remember the "play chew-chew" tip)
- no bad words
- extra perks that growing children need, especially DHA

For more on snacks, see page 145.

Just say no! You've successfully navigated the Garden of Eden without succumbing to too many temptations. Now you're at the checkout counter. You're surrounded with red-light foods appealingly presented at your child's eye level. The little mouth salivates

---

COMING SOON TO A SUPERMARKET NEAR YOU

NuVal is the name of a nutrition guidance system based on the Overall Nutritional Quality Index (ONQI) developed by Dr. David Katz, director of Yale University's Prevention Research Center, and a team of leading nutrition and public health experts throughout North America. The NuVal system factors in some thirty nutrients — both the good, such as antioxidants and fiber, and the bad, such as trans fat and added sugar — weights each based on its specific health effects, and translates all this into a single number between 1 and 100. The higher the number, the more nutritious the food. The system is currently being adopted by supermarket chains throughout the United States. For more information, visit www.NuVal.com. Also, for a fun and informative way to teach your kids how to become savvy supermarket shoppers, see www.NutritionDetectives.com.

---

and those eager hands are about to grab for the junk stuff (most of which contain all three bad words). Lovingly and convincingly you say, "We just don't eat that stuff in our family. I love you and I can't let you pollute your body and mind with that junk." Offer her one of the healthier treats she picked out instead.

10

Step 7: Supplements

While it's always best to get nutrients from real food, there may be circumstances when nutritional supplements are needed. Some children have erratic eating patterns. Also, because they grow so fast, kids need more nutrients per pound than adults do.

That said, remember supplements are just that — to be used *in addition to,* not instead of real food.

The most common nutrient deficiencies in kids are:

- calcium
- iodine
- iron
- magnesium
- omega-3 fats
- vitamin B-12
- vitamin C
- vitamin E
- zinc

HOW TO CHOOSE AN OMEGA-3 SUPPLEMENT

Many children are not fond of fish, and safe seafood is not always available to every family. An omega-3 supplement can correct this nutrient deficiency. Always choose an omega-3 supplement made from marine sources, not from plant sources such as flaxseed oil, as explained on page 108.

The two most important omega 3s are DHA and EPA. DHA is the most important omega 3 for the growing brain, and it is the one that has been most highly researched. EPA is also vital for the health of the immune system. So, either choose a DHA-only supplement or, if you choose one with DHA/EPA, select the formulation that contains DHA/EPA in around a 2:1 ratio — the same ratio of omega 3s that is found naturally in most wild salmon. While the USDA has yet to issue dietary guidelines for omega-3 supplements, the National Institutes of Health recommends 600 milligrams per day (DHA or DHA/EPA) per 2,000 calories.

Dosage of DHA.
- infants: at least 300 milligrams per day
- children two to three years: at least 400 milligrams per day
- children over four years, adults, and women who are pregnant or lactating: at least 600 milligrams per day

Source. Supplements come in three forms: oils by the teaspoon, capsules (such as soft gels), or soft chews. The favorite in our medical practice is Brainy Kidz, an individually wrapped fruit-based soft chew that children enjoy. The natural fruit flavor disguises any fishy taste. (See www.AskDrSears.com for omega-3 supplement sources.) You can also obtain a high-quality omega-3 salmon oil from www.VitalChoice.com.

SUSPECT SUPPLEMENTS

Use the same selection criteria for supplements that you would for other packaged foods, such as cereals. Avoid supplements that:

- display a cartoon character. What does SpongeBob know about the nutrients your child needs?
- have "bad words" on the ingredients list: high fructose corn syrup, number symbols (e.g., red #40), artificial sweeteners (e.g., aspartame, sucralose)

Safety. Look for the words Safe Source, which guarantee that every single batch of oil is third-party tested, certified for purity, and free of environmental contaminants, such as mercury, heavy metals, PCBs, and pesticides. There should be no "bad words" on the label. The formulation should be free of high fructose corn syrup and artificial colors and sweeteners.

MULTIVITAMINS: CHOOSING AND USING

If your child is going through a stage of erratic eating or grow-food refusals, your doctor may recommend a multivitamin/multimineral (MV/MM) preparation. Whether or not kids are helped by MV/MM supplements has been debated in medical journals for decades. Beware of well-meaning friends who tell you that science says MV/MM are not needed. Some "studies" suggesting supplements are useless are guilty of selective literature review, meaning they're biased toward one point of view.

A few years ago I chaired a scientific meeting on the topic "Do multivitamin/multimineral supplements really help children's health?" I put together a panel of children's nutrition experts, including two professors of nutrition from Harvard Medical School. All panel members were required to do a thorough review of the scientific studies to answer this question. Here are the conclusions of this panel, and of most nutritionists who know the medical studies:

Children who need a daily MV/MM to improve health and school performance:

- kids who have erratic eating patterns
- children in the lower socioeconomic demographic
- children eating a strict vegan diet
- children with intestinal disorders such as inflammatory bowel disease, celiac disease, or any illness that damages the absorptive abilities of the intestinal lining. Studies on these types of children show deficiencies in omega 3s, B-12, iron, magnesium, iodine, zinc, and folate.
- obese children. Many are iron-deficient.

Children who do not usually need a daily MV/MM. Kids who eat a steady diet of real foods rarely need supplements.

What to look for in a supplement. If you and your child's doctor believe your child needs an MV/MM supplement, there are certain things to look for. Each serving should contain at least 50 percent of the daily value that children need. This will be listed in the Supplement Facts table. (An exception to the 50 percent rule is the mineral calcium. Because calcium occupies so much room in a tablet, it is usually packaged separately as a calcium supplement rather than part of an MV/MM.)

Supplements should also be free of artificial sweeteners and food colorings.

III

Meal Plans and Recipes

*N*ow *that you know which foods can prevent NDD, in this section we will share with you meal plans and recipes that we personally use in our family and recommend in our pediatric practice. Children, like adults, prefer tasty fare. Most of these meal plans and recipes have been kid-tested in the Sears family kitchen. We wish to thank our daughter Hayden for supplying many of the recipes that she feeds our grandchildren. We hope you enjoy them.*

For more recipes and ways to feed your children grow foods, visit www.AskDrSears.com.

11

Nine Days of Sample Menus

These nine days of menus are given as a guide, and substitutions can easily be made. Note that we have added suggestions in parentheses for those who desire even more nutrients. Organic and free-range items should be used whenever possible. Peanuts should be avoided until age two. Honey should not be given to babies under one.

DAY 1

Breakfast

Whole wheat bagel with low-fat cream cheese or peanut butter or almond butter
Banana. Some kids may enjoy this sliced on their bagel.
Water or milk

Lunch

Lettuce roll: sliced turkey or chicken, tomato, and low-fat cream cheese rolled up or folded up in large leaves of romaine lettuce, like a burrito
Water or milk

Snack

Homemade pumpkin muffin (see recipe, page 202)
Small cup of 100 percent juice diluted with half water

Dinner

Healthy canned or homemade chili (low-fat varieties such as turkey, chicken, or vegetarian; add chunks of veggies or see recipe, page 190)
Homemade corn bread
Water or milk

Dessert

Frozen red grapes

DAY 2

Breakfast

Steel-cut oatmeal with cinnamon and fresh fruit and a little honey (or agave nectar) (see recipe, page 186)
Water or milk

Lunch

Bean and cheese burrito made with a whole wheat tortilla (add tomato or other cut-up veggies)
Small green salad with olive oil–based dressing (use dark greens such as spinach; add flaxseed oil)
Water or milk

Snack

Whole wheat crackers with peanut butter and honey
Small cup of 100 percent juice diluted with half water

Dinner

"Breakfast for dinner." Egg dishes are great for dinner. Try a veggie omelet.
Baked potato
Water or milk

Dessert

Small dish of berries with a dab of freshly made whipped cream on top

DAY 3

Breakfast

Whole-grain, low-in-sugar cereal with milk or soy milk (sprinkled with cinnamon and protein powder)
Large slice of melon
Water or milk

Lunch

Grilled cheese sandwich on whole wheat bread; use unprocessed
cheese (add tomato and avocado)
Large portion of carrot sticks, bell pepper loops, and broccoli
trees with hummus dip
Water or milk

Snack

Handful of nuts (walnuts, almonds — raw, add your own sea
salt)
Blueberries
Water or milk

Dinner

Lentil soup with vegetables (add flaxseed oil or salmon oil to each
serving, not while cooking) (see recipe, page 187)
Green salad with olive oil–based salad dressing (use dark greens
such as spinach; sprinkle with raw almonds instead of croutons;
use Corn and Black Bean Salsa recipe, page 189, as dressing)
Water or milk

Dessert

1/2 peach with a small scoop of vanilla frozen yogurt in the middle
(or low-fat plain yogurt sprinkled with a little agave nectar, cinnamon, and raw nuts)
Water or milk

DAY 4

Breakfast

Omelet made with favorite veggies (use DHA eggs)
Orange wedges
Water or milk

Lunch

Salad pita pocket. Fill half a whole wheat pita with salad made with
greens, diced veggies, cheese, and olive oil–based salad dressing
or hummus (use dark greens such as spinach or field greens)
Peach or other seasonal fresh fruit
Water or milk

Snack

String cheese
Apple slices
Water or milk

Dinner

Alaskan wild salmon with favorite sauce
Lightly steamed veggies
Wild or brown rice (or substitute quinoa)
Water or milk

Dessert

Homemade milkshake made with milk, frozen banana, and strawberries (add blueberries and some flaxseed oil)

DAY 5

Breakfast

Whole wheat blueberry pancakes with a dab of honey or freshly
made whipped cream on top (or agave nectar) (see page 184)
Milk or soy milk

Lunch

Tuna sandwich on whole wheat bread (add tomato and dark
lettuce)
Veggie sticks dipped in guacamole

Snack

Plain yogurt with fresh peaches and a dab of honey or agave nectar mixed together (add cinnamon)

Dinner

Taco salad made with greens, tomato, olives, kidney beans, and
cooked ground turkey sprinkled with tortilla chips and olive
oil–based dressing or salsa
Water or milk

Dessert

Homemade oatmeal-raisin cookie (use whole wheat flour; see
recipe, page 201)

DAY 6

Breakfast

Plain yogurt with granola or favorite whole-grain cereal mixed in
Grapes
Water or milk

Lunch

Quesadilla made with whole wheat tortilla (use low-fat cheese)
Guacamole and salsa to dip
Small green salad with olive oil–based salad dressing (use dark
   greens such as spinach)
Water or milk

Snack

Whole wheat toast with peanut butter
Water or milk

Dinner

Salmon on top of whole wheat pasta with marinara sauce
Large portion of veggies sautéed in olive oil and sprinkled with
   sea salt
Water or milk

Dessert

Sliced apples sprinkled with cinnamon

DAY 7

Breakfast

Smoothie (see recipe, pages 182–183)

Lunch

Pizza made on whole wheat English muffin or tortilla with veggies
on top
Melon
Water or milk

Snack

Tortilla chips and bean dip (add flaxseed or salmon oil to bean dip)
Small cup of 100 percent juice diluted with half water

Dinner

Whole wheat mac and cheese with chicken chunks mixed in
Large portion of veggies
Water or milk

Dessert

Smoothie popsicle from the leftover smoothie you made earlier
in the day

DAY 8

Breakfast

Yogurt parfait: plain yogurt with agave nectar or honey mixed in. Layer yogurt with berries and nutritious granola or whole-grain cereal.

Lunch

Peanut Butter Chicken Rice Bowl (see recipe, page 193)

Snack

Corn tortilla with Corn and Black Bean Salsa
Water or milk

Dinner

Salad dinner. Let your kids make their own salads with veggies, beans, nuts, sliced poultry, low-fat cheeses, or other creative leftovers
Water or milk

Dessert

Fresh or frozen berries in a wafer ice cream cone with a dab of freshly made whipped cream on top

DAY 9

Breakfast

Fruity French Toast (see recipe, page 184)
Water or milk

Lunch

Veggie kebabs, grilled or broiled
Whole wheat toast with favorite nut butter
Water or milk

Snack

Big slice of watermelon

Dinner

Lemony Rainbow Chicken (see recipe, page 192)
Green salad with olive oil–based dressing (use dark greens such as
    spinach)

Dessert

Pumpkin muffin

12

NDD-Prevention Recipes

Here are some of our favorite family recipes from the kitchens of Martha Sears and our daughter Hayden Sears-Livesay. These recipes are designed to be easily adjusted to fit each family's taste, and they can be altered to be gluten-free. Martha and Hayden like to cook large meals and keep the leftovers to use the next day. Enjoy!

BRAINY BREAKFASTS

DR. BILL'S SCHOOL-ADE SMOOTHIE

We have been making this Sears family recipe an average of five days a week for the past ten years. Our whole family enjoys it, as do the families in our pediatric practice. It is one of our top "prescriptions" in the NDD-prevention plan.

Serves 4–5

Ingredients

2 *cups Greek-style organic yogurt, plain, nonfat*

2–3 *cups organic milk, soy beverage, or pomegranate or vegetable or fruit juice (e.g., carrot, greens; grape juice works especially well)*

1 *cup frozen blueberries*

1 *cup mixed frozen fruit (e.g., strawberries, mango, papaya, or pineapple)*

1 *banana*

2 *tbsp. ground flaxseeds*

4 *ounces tofu*

1 *tbsp. cinnamon*

2 *tbsp. nonhydrogenated peanut butter*

Optional Add-ins

2 *servings whey protein powder*

1–2 *servings multivitamin/multimineral chocolate- or vanilla-flavored powder (See www.AskDrSears.com for the brand we recommend.)*

¼ *cup raisins or dates (for extra sweetness and fiber)*

2 *kiwis (for extra vitamin C)*

2 *tbsp. wheat germ*

1 *cup fresh baby spinach leaves*

2 *tbsp. pomegranate seeds (available in the refrigerated section of nutrition stores)*

Combine all the ingredients and blend until smooth. Add more liquid to get the desired consistency. Blend again. Serve immediately, before the air settles and while the mixture has a bubbly milkshake texture.

FRUITY FRENCH TOAST

This version of a family favorite is so yummy, there is no need to add syrup on top!

Serves 4–6

Ingredients

6 eggs, beaten
1 tbsp. vanilla
⅓ cup thawed orange juice or pineapple juice concentrate (from the freezer section — do not dilute)
1 tbsp. extra virgin olive oil
About 6 slices of whole wheat bread

Optional Toppings

Top with cinnamon, berries, whipped cream, or agave nectar, or spread with nut butter.

Mix all the ingredients together except the bread and oil. Heat the oil in a skillet. Soak the bread in the egg mixture and carefully place it in the skillet. Brown on both sides and serve.

CINNAMON APPLE OR BLUEBERRY PANCAKES

Adding nutritious foods into this kid-favorite breakfast makes it a healthy start.

16 four-inch pancakes

Ingredients

2 cups whole-grain pancake mix
1¾ cups milk or buttermilk
2 eggs
¼ cup honey or fresh apple juice
1 tbsp. ground cinnamon (or more, to taste)
½ cup ground whole-grain fiber (e.g., oatbran, etc.)
⅓ cup whipping cream

1 cup finely chopped apple (or blueberries)
¼ cup ground flaxseeds

Optional Toppings
*Instead of maple syrup, top with this homemade applesauce. Puree
2–3 apples with one ripe banana and a little cinnamon in a
food processor.*

Mix the pancake mix, buttermilk, eggs, honey or juice, and
cinnamon in a bowl and blend until smooth. Add the fiber
grains and whipping cream and blend lightly. Stir in the
chopped apple or blueberries and ground flaxseeds.

YUMMY YOGURT PARFAIT
This luscious-looking dish can be served for breakfast, lunch, or
dessert.

Serves 2–3

Ingredients
1½ cups Greek-style organic yogurt, plain, nonfat
½ cup granola
½ cup blueberries
½ cup strawberries
1 tsp. slivered almonds
1 tsp. cinnamon

Optional Add-in
Agave nectar (to sweeten yogurt)

Place ½ of the yogurt in two or three cute clear glasses.
Sprinkle in half of the granola and one of the fruits. Then
add the rest of the yogurt. Place the rest of the granola on
top and add the other fruit (place the child's favorite fruit
on top). Add the almonds and sprinkle cinnamon on top.

THE TASTIEST, HEALTHIEST, MOST AWESOME OATMEAL

Steel-cut oatmeal has more nutrients than regular rolled oats.

Serves 3–4

Ingredients
1 cup steel-cut oatmeal
4 cups water
¼ cup ground flaxseeds

Optional Toppings
Add cinnamon, plain organic nonfat yogurt, berries, or nuts.

Before bedtime, place the oats and water in a Crock Pot and set to heat on low overnight. In the morning, add the flaxseed. Serve with your favorite topping. (If you don't have a Crock Pot, just follow the directions on the box.)

LUSCIOUS LUNCHES

VERY GOOD VEGGIE SANDWICH

Ingredients
Whole-grain bread
Canola oil mayonnaise
Favorite mustard or salad dressing
Avocado slices
Tomato slices
Veggies: broccoli, radishes, alfalfa sprouts, etc.
Sunflower seeds (grind for young children to avoid choking)

Optional Add-ins
Spinach leaves
Hard-boiled egg slices

Spread bread with mayo and mustard or salad dressing, then pile on the remaining ingredients. Let the kids stack the veggies.

BUTTERNUT SQUASH LENTIL SOUP
Yum, Yum! Get the kiddos to help chop!

Serves 4–6

Ingredients
2 tbsp. extra virgin olive oil
1 onion
3 cloves garlic, crushed
2 celery stalks, diced
4 tbsp. curry powder
8 cups chicken or vegetable broth
1 14.5-ounce can fire-roasted crushed tomatoes
2 cups chopped butternut squash
3 sliced carrots
2½ cups dry lentils (any color; I especially like red for this recipe)
Sea salt and pepper

Optional Add-ins
Fresh basil, sprinkled as a garnish
Red pepper flakes. For more spice, add to individual bowls.

Heat the oil in a large pot and sauté onions, garlic, and celery for about 3 minutes. Add the remaining ingredients and bring the mixture to a boil. Simmer for about 15 minutes.

Be careful not to overcook; the vegetables should stay a little firm so they maintain more of their nutrients. Add salt and pepper to taste. Leftovers are GREAT!!!

DR. BILL'S TUNA OR SALMON SALAD

This tuna or salmon salad truly meets our definition of a nutrient-dense food. And it's so tasty, every family member will enjoy it.

Serves 2–3

Ingredients

8 ounces tuna or salmon fillet, fresh or fresh-frozen* (or canned)
2 chopped hard-boiled eggs
¼ cup diced dill pickle
⅓–½ cup canola oil mayonnaise
1 tbsp. Dijon mustard
¼ cup sunflower seeds
1 tbsp. lemon juice
1 tsp. minced garlic or onion (or to taste)
½ tsp. ground pepper
½ tsp. dried dill weed
1 tbsp. olive oil
¼ cup chopped tomato
Whole wheat pita or tortilla
½ cup bean sprouts, broccoli, or alfalfa sprouts

Optional Add-ins

1–2 tbsp. fresh red chili peppers
1 tbsp. hummus

---

*See www.AskDrSears.com for my favorite seafood sources.

Grill, bake, or poach the fillet. Chop it into small pieces or flake it with a fork. Mix it in a bowl with the other ingredients except the pita and sprouts. Chill the salad and serve it in a pita pocket or burrito-style on a warmed whole wheat tortilla. Garnish it with sprouts. For added nutrition and taste, spread a layer of hummus on the bread first.

CORN AND BLACK BEAN SALSA

This dish is really more like pico de gallo than salsa. We keep some in the refrigerator and add it to so many things! If any ingredient on our list is "icky" in your house, go ahead and skip it.

About 3 cups

Ingredients
1 can black beans (drain about half of the juice)
1 cup corn (thawed frozen corn or cut off the cob)
½ cup diced water chestnuts
¼ cup extra virgin olive oil
1½ tbsp. apple cider vinegar
1 tsp. ground cumin
¼ cup diced cilantro
Splash of hot sauce or Tabasco (or to taste)
Hummus (mix in a scoop for a creamy consistency)
Salt and pepper to taste
½ cup diced tomato
1 avocado, chopped into chunks

Mix all of the ingredients except the tomatoes and avocado and chill. (It tastes best when it is chilled overnight.) When ready to serve, add the tomato and avocado.

DELICIOUS DINNERS

MARTHA'S THREE-BEAN CHILI (VEGETARIAN OR CHICKEN)
This nutrient-dense meal introduces kids to healthy spices and a variety of beans.

Serves 8–10

Ingredients
1 tbsp. canola oil
1 onion, chopped
1 clove garlic, minced
16 ounces firm tofu, cubed or crumbled or 1 pound boneless chicken breast, chopped
1 15-ounce can kidney beans, drained
1 15-ounce can garbanzo beans, drained
1 15-ounce can pinto beans, drained
1 tbsp. chili powder (or to taste)
1 tbsp. sea salt (or to taste)
1 tsp. ground cumin
20 ounces tomato sauce
1 tbsp. molasses
2 tbsp. unsweetened cocoa

Optional Add-ins (for more spice)
2 tsp. paprika
¾ tsp. cayenne pepper
¼ tsp. turmeric
¼ tsp. ground coriander
¼ tsp. ground cardamom

Sauté the onions and garlic in the oil. Add the tofu or chicken and sauté until cooked through. Add the remaining ingredients and bring to a boil. Simmer for two hours. Serve with corn bread.

DR. PETER SEARS'S HEALTHY CHICKEN NUGGETS

After handling raw chicken, wash your hands with soap and water before touching other surfaces or handling other foods.

About 15 chicken nuggets

Ingredients

1 pound organic, hormone-free boneless, skinless chicken breasts
1½ teaspoons sea salt
1 omega-3-enriched egg
2 cups all-purpose flour
2 cups regular or whole wheat bread crumbs

Optional Add-ins

1½ teaspoons black pepper
8 tablespoons ricotta cheese (for creamier texture)

Preheat the oven to 375°. Cut the chicken breasts into roughly 2-inch by 2-inch cubes and place in the food processor. And add sea salt and pepper (optional). If using ricotta cheese, add it to the food processor along with the chicken. Pulse all the ingredients until the mixture is of even consistency (it only takes a few seconds). Set up a dredging station with a plate containing flour, a bowl containing the beaten egg, and a plate containing bread crumbs. Form the chicken mixture into about 2-inch by 1½-inch nugget-size pieces. Coat one nugget at a time lightly in flour, dip it into the beaten egg, shake off the excess egg, and then roll it in bread crumbs (dip fingers into water in between nuggets to prevent fingers from sticking to nuggets). Place the nuggets on a cookie sheet that has been lightly coated with olive oil. Bake for 8 to 10 minutes on each side or until the chicken is cooked through and the juices run clear. Serve along with your favorite veggies and/or other healthy side dish!

LEMONY RAINBOW CHICKEN 🗸

This one-dish meal can be custom-fitted to your family's tastes and nutritional needs. It can also be made vegan or gluten- or dairy-free. Serve leftovers on top of a bed of fresh spinach or in a whole wheat pita pocket for lunch the next day. This dish goes great with a green side salad.

Serves 4–6

Ingredients
2 tbsp. extra virgin olive oil
1 onion, chopped
3–4 cloves garlic, crushed
2 cups dry quinoa
4 cups free-range chicken broth or organic vegetable broth
3 chicken breasts or tofu cut into 1-inch pieces
½ cup lemon juice or the juice from 3 lemons (add zest if desired)
Sea salt and pepper to taste
Rainbow of veggies: 3–4 cups of your family's favorite veggies,
*   chopped. Our favorite rainbow:*
*   Red: red bell pepper*
*   Orange: shredded carrot*
*   Yellow: yellow bell pepper*
*   Green: zucchini*
*   Blue: handful of dried blueberries*
*   Purple: purple onion*
*   1 cup finely chopped basil leaves*

Optional Add-ins
½ cup sliced raw almonds
Parmesan cheese, grated
Red pepper flakes

In a large pot, heat the oil and sauté the onions and garlic. Add the quinoa, broth, and chicken. Bring to a boil and cover. Reduce heat to low and simmer for 15 minutes. Add the lemon juice and salt and pepper. Stir in your rainbow of veggies and the basil. Replace the lid for a couple minutes. Stir in the almonds and Parmesan cheese, and sprinkle with red pepper flakes at the end for some kick if desired.

~~PEANUT~~ Nut BUTTER CHICKEN RICE BOWLS

Your family will love the taste of their beloved peanut butter, as it stars in this delicious and nutritious dish. This dish goes great with a green side salad.

Serves 4–6

Ingredients
Sauce
4 tbsp. creamy or chunky nonhydrogenated peanut butter (or any other nut butter), without added sugar
3 tbsp. soy sauce or Bragg Liquid Aminos
½ cup 100 percent apple juice (more if you like it thinner)
2 tsp. lemon juice
Hot sauce to taste

1 tbsp. extra virgin olive oil
3 chicken breasts cut into bite-size pieces
3 cups of your family's favorite vegetables, chopped into bite-size pieces. We use red and yellow bell peppers, broccoli, onions, zucchini, and mushrooms.

1 tbsp. soy sauce or Bragg Liquid Aminos
1 cup brown or wild rice or quinoa, cooked according to directions on the box

Mix together the peanut butter, soy sauce, and apple juice
in a small saucepan. Add the lemon juice and hot sauce.
Heat oil in a large skillet or wok and sauté the chicken until
just cooked. Remove the chicken and add the vegetables plus
the soy sauce. Sauté until the vegetables are cooked but still
firm. Mix the chicken back in. Serve the chicken and vegetable mixture over rice in bowls. Heat the peanut sauce
briefly. Spoon the sauce over each bowl or let each person
add their own sauce.

TUNA OR SALMON CAKES

This meal is full of protein, and you can make it in a jiffy. Be creative and come up with your own flavor!! These are great served
on top of a green salad or steamed spinach.

Serves about 2

Ingredients

1 6-ounce can light chunk tuna, drained or canned wild or Alaskan
   salmon
2 eggs
¼ cup whole wheat bread crumbs (you can skip these if you want,
   but they help the cakes stick together)
1 clove garlic, crushed or ¼ tsp. granulated garlic (not garlic salt)
2 tsp. olive oil

Optional Add-ins

Mexican: 3 tbsp. corn, 3 tbsp. black beans, dash of hot sauce or
   Tabasco (or just add about ½ cup Corn and Black Bean Salsa)
Asian: 1 tbsp. soy sauce, 3 tbsp. peas, 3 tbsp. shredded carrots

*Italian: 2 tbsp. marinara or pizza sauce, 2 tbsp. diced bell peppers,
   1 tbsp. diced black olives, mozzarella cheese sprinkled on top*
Thai: 1 tsp. curry power, 3 tbsp. shredded zucchini

Mix all the ingredients together. Heat the oil in a skillet.
Place 3 or 4 scoops of the mixture in a skillet and flatten
them to about ½ inch. Brown on both sides.

FISH STICKS YOUR WAY!

Ditch the junky store-bought fish sticks and whip up your own,
using Alaskan or wild fish. Salmon works *great!* Make a double
batch and freeze some for a quick meal or snack.

Serves 3–4

Ingredients

½ cup whole wheat flour or corn flour or oat flour
*1 cup whole wheat bread crumbs or cracker crumbs (make your
   own with heels of bread)*
1 tbsp. granulated garlic (not garlic salt)
2 tsp. sea salt
½ tsp. stevia (or substitute brown sugar)
3–4 fish fillets
2 eggs, beaten
Olive oil

Optional Add-ins

⅓ cup Parmesan cheese
Curry powder
Red pepper flakes
*Fresh minced parsley or cilantro (or any other mixed seasoning
   that your family enjoys)*

Preheat the oven to 375°. Mix all of the dry ingredients in a large Ziploc or other plastic bag. Cut the fish fillets into strips that are at least 1 inch thick. Put the fish strips into another bowl with the beaten eggs. Carefully transfer each piece of fish to the bag with the dry mix. Seal the bag and carefully roll it around, gently coating the fish. (Hint: If the adults want more flavor or spice, do half the fish and then add some more seasonings to the bag and do the other half.) Transfer each piece of fish onto a lightly oiled cookie sheet or baking tray. Flip each piece of fish over so that both sides have a little olive oil on them. Bake for 8–10 minutes.

Serve the fish sticks with lightly steamed veggies. Skip the ketchup and instead try marinara sauce, hummus, guacamole, a squeeze of lemon juice, or the peanut butter sauce from the Peanut Butter Chicken Rice Bowls recipe, page 193.

SWEET POTATO FRIES

A delicious, nutritious alternative to store-bought fries.

Serves 4–6

Ingredients
4–6 sweet potatoes
3 tbsp. olive oil
Sea salt to taste

Optional Toppings
Sprinkle with granulated garlic or grated Parmesan cheese before serving.

Preheat oven to 450°. Wash and slice sweet potatoes into wedges about ½ inch thick. Toss with olive oil and salt. Place potatoes in a single layer on a cookie sheet. Bake for

15 minutes. Flip the wedges over and bake for 15 more minutes or until lightly browned.

FISH IN A BAG
Make fantastic fish fillets.

Serves 4

Ingredients
¼ cup olive oil
1 tbsp. lemon pepper seasoning
1 tbsp. fresh-squeezed lemon juice
1–2 tsp. dill weed, fresh or dried
1–2 tsp. fennel seeds
1–2 tsp. soy sauce
3 6-ounce fillets of salmon, tuna, or halibut

Optional Add-ins
Garlic, crushed (to taste)
Fresh ginger, grated (to taste)
Brown sugar

In a large bowl, combine all the ingredients except the fillets and mix well. Cut the fish into strips about the size of your pinky. Place the marinade and fish in a large Ziploc bag, close carefully, and turn it until all the pieces are evenly coated. Refrigerate for an hour or more. Place the marinated strips on a baking rack under a broiler for around five minutes. *Don't overcook!* The fish is done when it flakes easily with a fork.

SUPERSNACKS

DR. BILL'S NUTTY-FRUITY TRAIL MIX

Raw nuts provide a wonderful source of brain-building fats. *Caution:* Nuts and seeds pose a choking hazard to children under three or four years of age.

2½ cups; 1 serving = 1 palmful

Ingredients
½ cup raw almonds
½ cup raw walnuts
⅓ cup raw pecans
⅓ cup raw pistachio nuts
¼ cup raw sunflower seeds
⅓ cup raw pumpkin seeds
⅓ cup raisins
⅓ cup dried cranberries or tart cherries

Optional Add-ins
Other nuts your child prefers
Soy nuts
Unsweetened carob chips
A few semisweet chocolate chips

Encourage your child to scoop each of these ingredients out of their packages into a bowl and toss them together in the bowl. Place ½ cup in individual baggies for away-from-home snacks. If your family is not used to eating raw nuts, use some raw and some roasted nuts.

NUTBUTTER BALLS

Our kids love these tasty "balls" for a snack as well as for dessert.
Let your kids help you roll them into balls or other fun shapes.

30 small balls

Ingredients
½ *cup carob powder*
½ *cup honey*
½ *cup peanut butter*
½ *cup raw sunflower seeds*
½ *cup sesame seeds*
½ *cup oats or quinoa flakes*
Shredded coconut

Optional Add-ins
¼–½ *cup flaxseed meal*
Diced raisins or dates

Mix together by hand all the ingredients except the coconut. Form the batter into bite-size balls and roll them in the coconut.

HEALTHY GRANOLA BARS

This recipe was created by a mother in our practice, Alisa Langevin, for her children with nut and egg allergies.

12–15 bars

Ingredients
2 *cups rolled oats, ground in a food processor*
½ *cup wheat germ, unsweetened*
⅛ *cup flaxseed meal*
2 *cups brown rice cereal or Rice Krispies*
1 *cup nonfat dry milk*
½ *tsp. cinnamon*

1 tsp. salt
¾ cup canola oil
½ cup honey
½ cup pure maple syrup
2 tsp. vanilla
¼ cup chocolate chips

Preheat the oven to 300°. Grease a 13 x 9 cookie sheet. In a medium bowl combine the oats, wheat germ, flaxseed meal, rice cereal, dry milk, cinnamon, and salt. Mix in the oil, honey, syrup, vanilla, and chocolate chips. Be sure there are no dry, powdery areas remaining. The mixture will be granular.

Press the mixture evenly onto the cookie sheet. Press down to distribute the mixture into the corners of the cookie sheet. Bake 18–20 minutes or until the outer edges turn brown. Remove from the oven and let sit for 30 minutes to set and cool. Cut into squares. Keep refrigerated.

DELIGHTFUL DESSERTS

DELICIOUS GELATO

A Sears family favorite, this recipe was sent to us by Debbie Puente, who learned this technique from Sicilian chef Ciccio Sultano. It couldn't be easier, and the fresh peach flavor is astonishing. The texture should be somewhere between soft-serve ice cream and dense, chewy traditional gelato. Depending on the sweetness of your peaches, you may want to add more sugar.

Serves 6–8

Ingredients
3 pounds peaches, peeled and pitted
¼ cup sugar (or more to taste)
½ cup mascarpone, crème fraîche, or yogurt

Cut the peaches into very small pieces. The smaller you cut them, the faster they will freeze and the finer the final texture will be. Arrange the peach pieces in a single layer on a rimmed cookie sheet and freeze solid, about 2 hours.

Put the frozen peach pieces in a food processor with the sugar and grind briefly. Add the mascarpone, crème fraîche, or yogurt and pulse until the mixture is smooth.

Empty the contents of the food processor into a container and freeze again, 20 to 30 minutes, before serving. If the ice cream freezes solid, simply process it briefly again before serving.

DR. BILL'S JIFFY GELATO

Place a 6-to-8-ounce cup of organic plain Greek-style yogurt in the freezer for 45 minutes. When it is soft-frozen, stir in your favorite additions, such as slivered almonds and blueberries, or just add honey.

Serves 1

OUTSTANDING OATMEAL-RAISIN COOKIES

Encourage your kids to help you bake this tasty snack or dessert.

2 dozen

Ingredients
½ cup honey
*½ cup grapeseed oil, canola oil, or butter or 8 ounces silken-soft
   tofu*
½ tsp. baking soda

1 tbsp. ground cinnamon
1 tsp. vanilla
¼ tsp. baking powder
¼ tsp. sea salt
1 egg
1½ cups oats or granola
1 cup whole wheat pastry flour or ⅓ cup almond meal and
⅔ cup flour
1 cup raisins

Optional Add-ins
½ cup chopped walnuts
½ cup carob chips

Preheat the oven to 375°. Combine all the ingredients except the oats, flour, and raisins, and mix thoroughly. Stir in the oats, flour, and raisins. Drop the batter by teaspoonfuls on a cookie sheet and bake for approximately 10 minutes or until cookies are a light brown.

STICKY PUMPKIN MUFFINS

Pumpkin is not only yummy for little tummies, it is packed with nutrients. You can make these plain or try the add-ins for a more interesting flavor.

About 1 dozen

Ingredients
1 cup whole wheat flour (use brown rice flour for gluten-free)
½ cup oat flour
1–2 tsp. cinnamon
1 tsp. nutmeg
1 tsp. sea salt
2 tsp. baking soda

2 eggs
½ cup 100 percent orange juice concentrate, thawed (do not dilute)
½ cup pure maple syrup
1 tsp. stevia (or brown sugar)
2 tbsp. honey or agave nectar
2 tsp. vanilla extract
1 cup canned 100 percent pumpkin

Optional Add-ins
Dried cranberries
Raisins
Nuts
Coconut
½ cup carrots, grated
½ zucchini, grated (Hint: for really picky eaters who won't eat green things no matter how small, thinly shave off the green peel before grating, so that the zucchini becomes invisible.)

Preheat the oven to 350°. Mix the dry ingredients in one bowl and the wet ingredients in another. Add the dry mixture to the wet mixture. Include any add-ins that you desire. Fill greased muffin tins three-quarters full and bake for 30–40 minutes. Cool completely.

Index